BACK Rx

BACK Rx

A FIFTEEN-MINUTE-A-DAY
YOGA- AND PILATES-BASED PROGRAM
TO END LOW BACK PAIN

Vijay Vad, M.D.

and Hilary Hinzmann

GOTHAM
BOOKS

GOTHAM BOOKS
Published by Penguin Group (USA) Inc.
375 Hudson Street, New York, New York 10014, U.S.A.
Penguin Books Ltd, Registered Offices: 80 Strand, London WC2R 0RL, England
Penguin Books Australia Ltd, 250 Camberwell Road, Camberwell, Victoria 3124, Australia
Penguin Books Canada Ltd, 10 Alcorn Avenue, Toronto, Ontario, Canada M4V 3B2
Penguin Books (NZ) Ltd, Cnr Rosedale and Airborne Roads, Albany Auckland 1310, New Zealand

Published by Gotham Books, a division of Penguin Group (USA) Inc.
First printing, January 2004
10 9 8 7 6

Gotham Books and the skyscraper logo are trademarks of Penguin Group (USA) Inc.

LIBRARY OF CONGRESS CATALOGING-IN-PUBLICATION DATA
Vad, Vijay.
   Back RX : a fifteen-minute-a-day yoga- and Pilates-based program to end low back pain / Vijay Vad,
      and Hilary Hinzmann.
      p. cm.
   Includes bibliographical references.
   ISBN 1-592-40045-0 (alk. paper)
   1. Pilates method. 2. Backache—Alternative treatment. 3. Yoga. I. Hinzmann, Hillary. II. Title.

RA781.V23 2004
617.5'6406—dc22   2003049337

Printed in the United States of America
Set in Electra
Designed by Tina Thompson

To my beautiful wife, Dilshaad, whose struggle with back pain motivated me to find a solution; to my parents, Drs. Bal and Lata Vad, who are my greatest supporters, friends, and mentors; and to all the low back pain sufferers in the world—may this book help you regain full quality of life.

VV

Contents

Acknowledgments

We would like to thank Chris Godek, whose knowledge and insight guided us through this project; our agent, Stuart Krichevsky, for his unfailing support, diligence, and wisdom; J. B. Berns, for helping to design the exercise programs, and Tara Parker-Pope, who first suggested the need for this book.

At Gotham Books we have had the benefit of a wonderful group of publishers; thanks especially to William Shinker, Lauren Marino, Erin Moore, Sabrina Bowers, and Gary Perkinson for helping us to fulfill our vision for the book. Thanks also to McLain Bennett for her work on the photographs and to Tina Thompson for her design of the book.

Introduction:

The Back Rx Way to a Healthy, Pain-Free Back

If you're reading this book, you're probably all too familiar with the pain of a low back injury. A strained muscle in the low back can make you gasp with pain at the slightest movement. The herniation of a spinal disk, the most troublesome cause of severe low back pain, can virtually cripple you. Worst of all, in the aftermath of a low back injury, pain may take up permanent residence almost anywhere in the back or legs, including sites far removed from the point of injury.

If you're hurting now, skip ahead to page xvii for some simple ways to ease the pain. Come back to read these pages when you're feeling better. In order to make a full and lasting recovery from low back pain, you must first understand what causes it.

In North America, four out of five people will suffer a serious episode of low back pain at some point in their lives. Only the common cold causes more lost work days than low back pain for adults under forty-five years of age.

Low back injuries usually heal within weeks, a testament to the back's inherent strength and resilience. But long-term healing is notoriously difficult to achieve. One episode of low back pain generally leads to another. Four out of five people will suffer a recurrence within one year, and then face a 70–80% risk of further recurrences. The right treatment can make all the difference between healing completely, building a more injury-resistant and resilient back in the process, and falling into a downward spiral of recurrent injury that defeats every measure of conventional and alternative care and leads to failed back syndrome, long-term dependency on pain medication, and even surgery. That downward spiral traps far too many low back pain sufferers.

I've had to heal my own low back pain. So I write this book both as a physician and as a fellow sufferer. The Back Rx program enabled me to beat my low back pain for good. And it has helped thousands of patients I see in my sports medicine practice and research at the Hospital for Special Surgery, an affiliate of Cornell University Medical Center in New York, where I also serve on the faculty as a professor. Back Rx achieves these results by blending carefully selected elements of rehabilitation, yoga, and Pilates with a central focus on breath control. It is one of the few exercise programs for the low back to be shown effective in controlled clinical trials.

In an ongoing study, my research colleagues and I are monitoring the progress of two groups of low back patients who receive the same medical care and take the same pain medication, except that one group does the Back Rx program for fifteen minutes three times a week. At the end of the first year, the group doing Back Rx had a 70% success/cure rate (as measured by a more than 50% reduction in low back pain), whereas the other group had only a 33% success/cure rate. The group doing Back Rx also needed much less pain medication and had significantly less recurrence of back pain than the other group.

Building on the work of many other low back pain researchers and clinicians at the Hospital for Special Surgery and elsewhere, my research and clinical practice have demonstrated that an exercise program like Back Rx can be the key to healing low back pain without surgery or long-term dependence on medication.

My patients come from every walk of life, including professional sports, which allows me to see the full range of low back problems. Professional athletes are especially interesting patients in this regard. Understanding why even highly conditioned individuals are susceptible to low back pain provides great insight into the common denominators of this baffling medical condition and how best to address them.

I see professional athletes as private patients and in my role as a consulting physician for the ATP tennis tour and the PGA golf tour. My involvement with both tours began with research studies whose results provide powerful evidence for the effectiveness of the Back Rx program. I initiated this research in 1999–2000, when I spent a year on the road with the ATP tennis tour.

During my year on tour with the ATP, I had two main jobs to do. One was to find qualified low back care physicians in the tour's many stops around the world, from Tashkent, Uzbekistan, to Moscow, Russia, to Rome, Italy, to Tokyo, Japan, to Shanghai, China. The other was to conduct a research study into why low back pain is so prevalent among professional tennis players.

The study I conducted found that the players most susceptible to low back pain had the least range of motion in the hips. In 2001 the PGA asked me to do a parallel study of professional golfers. This study produced the same results, showing a significant link between a restricted range of motion in the hips and the incidence of low back pain.

This finding is important for the rest of us, whether we are fitter than average or committed couch potatoes, because of the sedentary nature of modern life and work. Sitting in chairs, which most of us do for long hours every day at work, school, and home, leads inexorably to a restricted range of motion in the hips.

The Back Rx program accordingly features exercises specifically designed to counteract this tendency and increase the range of motion in the hips.

The treatment room at a professional golf or tennis match is a microcosm of the low back pain world. On one table a top-10 player may be receiving treatment from an acupuncturist, while different competitors work with chiropractors, massage therapists, and osteopaths, as well as specialists in conventional physical therapy and rehabilitative medicine. I have observed that although no single one of these therapies works for everyone, each of them works for large numbers of people. Back Rx incorporates insights and healing knowledge from all of them, and in the course of the book I will offer guidelines for choosing which treatments are best suited to your own individual needs.

One thing that everyone who studies and treats low back pain agrees on is that it is fundamentally a mind-body problem. As we'll see in more detail in Chapter 2, emotional factors and psychological stress play a major role in the onset and persistence of low back pain.

A number of books have emphasized the mind's role in low back pain in a conceptual way, without offering reliable, concrete methods for putting the concept to practical use. The way one recent book puts it is typical: to heal low back pain, it tells readers vaguely, "learn to work with your negative feelings." Negative feelings from stressful experiences can indeed hinder full recovery and heighten recurrences. But healing low back pain begins not with psychotherapy, but with mind-body physiotherapy. You have to engage the mind at the fundamental level of body awareness, posture, and balance first. These three fundamentals form the essential foundation for healing the whole person.

Back Rx meets this challenge and teaches you how to engage the mind in healing through its focus on breath control, a key feature of both yoga and Pilates.

In my sports medicine and back care practice, my research on low back pain, and my own efforts to lead a healthy lifestyle, I've gained an increasing appreciation for the benefits of yoga and Pilates. Yoga, which I first learned to do at my grandfather's side as a young child in India, engages the entire body in healthy breathing, while freeing the mind to focus without distraction or anxiety on anything it needs to do. This age-old practice has a mind-body potential that the latest neuroscience is only beginning to understand. For its part Pilates, whose founder, Joseph Pilates, was greatly influenced by his study of yoga, is the best strengthening practice yet developed for the core body muscles—of the torso, back, abdomen, pelvis, and thighs—that are crucial to good back health.

The paradox is that although yoga and Pilates are ultimately the best possible way to maximize back health, in the short run the vigorous twists, turns, and bends of advanced yoga and Pilates can actually cause back injuries. It's quite a catch-22: the very thing that can help you the most can very easily hurt you.

Back Rx solves this problem with a carefully sequenced introduction of yoga- and Pilates-based movements and poses that will strengthen the back without traumatizing it. From the first step on, this sequence of medical yoga and medical Pilates addresses the body and mind together by showing you how to find and follow your natural breathing rhythm. The slow, sustained, deep, gentle breathing of Back Rx helps you in two ways. It automatically clears and refocuses the mind, and thus begins to melt away emotional and mental stress without any direct mental effort or concentration. And it tunes the body, so that each deepening breath progressively relaxes and conditions injured or atrophied muscles.

There are three series of Back Rx exercises to heal and strengthen your back. Each series takes fifteen minutes to complete and should be done three times a week for eight weeks on average. Series A alone will get you moving pain-free again after an acute low back injury. Many patients maintain good long-term back health by continuing to do Series A regularly, without moving on to Series B or C.

For those who want to raise their back fitness for sports and recreational enjoyment or as a stress-, injury-, and age-fighter, however, Series B offers a vigorous back toning routine and Series C provides a strenuous core body workout.

The vast majority of low back pain sufferers, more than 80%, can heal with Back Rx alone. For the small percentage who need to take other measures as well, Back Rx can be the spine that holds an effective treatment program together. There are exciting developments that can minimize the invasiveness and maximize the benefits of back treatments and surgeries. I look forward to telling you about them later in the book, including some minimally invasive, nonsurgical procedures that I have been fortunate enough to help innovate.

The Back Rx prescription offers a comprehensive mind-body solution for the mind-body problem of low back pain. Its combination of the most advanced modern medicine with the ancient wisdom of yoga and the core strengthening of Pilates will empower you to take your healing into your own hands and become your own best physician. The ancient yogists calculated that a human being takes 21,600 breaths a day, and the goal of yoga is to make every single breath a completely healthy one. If you can incorporate Back Rx into your life, you'll make a great start at reaching that goal and living pain-free.

LOW BACK PAIN FIRST AID CHEST

What to Do if You're in Pain Right Now

After a low back injury, follow these simple steps to ease your pain and begin your healing.

- Focus on and regulate your breathing. Proper breathing in a slow, controlled rhythm is the fastest pain reliever you can use. It shifts the mind's attention away from the pain and triggers the body's natural relaxation response. You can do this in any position, but if possible:
  - Lie flat on the floor on your back with your knees up and your lower legs resting on a chair, an ottoman, or some pillows, or lie on your side in bed in a fetal position with a pillow between your knees. These positions should take the strain off your lower back, but if another position feels better, that's fine. Every injury is different. Let your body guide you into the least painful position possible.
  - Slow your breathing down as much as possible. Exhale fully, then inhale deeply and hold the breath in your lungs for a count of three. Exhale fully, and continue breathing in this way for at least two to three minutes.
  - Repeat this process throughout the day to calm yourself and to deliver extra oxygen to overstressed muscles and disks, allowing them to begin to relax, breathe, and take in nourishment.
- Use visual imagery to guide your breathing and enhance the relaxation response. For example, try imagining your breath as a wave of golden light flowing through your entire body. Another good technique is to picture yourself in a favorite spot, real or imagined, where you feel safe and at ease.

  The more relaxed your breathing becomes, the less pain you will feel. As you become better able to focus on your breathing for a few minutes at a time, you will also prepare your mind and body to work together in the rest of your healing.
- Pain ≠ Gain. Being overly stoic may actually slow your recovery. Take anti-inflammatory and pain-relief medication to speed healing.
  - The most readily available over-the-counter pain relief medicines are aspirin, ibuprofen (Advil), and acetaminophen (Tylenol). Ibuprofen is

generally the best choice for low back pain, because unlike acetaminophen, it combines pain relief and anti-inflammatory benefits.

- Liquid gel pills work best, because they are absorbed more readily in the bloodstream. As a general rule, unless a doctor prescribes otherwise, you should take two liquid gel ibuprofen two to three times a day.

- Everybody reacts to medicine slightly differently, and you may find that it helps to to combine ibuprofen with acetaminophen, taking the first for pain and inflammation and the second for additional pain relief. In any case, do not take more than eight pills a day, total, unless your doctor prescribes otherwise.

- People with diabetes should be especially careful not to take high doses of these medicines for extended periods, because of the potential for kidney damage. Anti-inflammatory medication is also contraindicated for those with a history of gastric ulcers or compromised kidney function.

- If severe pain persists after seven to ten days of taking ibuprofen and/or acetaminophen, you should consult a physician.

- If over-the-counter medicines don't lessen your pain and inflammation significantly, don't wait a whole week to go to the doctor. More powerful pain relievers, anti-inflammatories, and muscle relaxants are available by prescription, and they are safe if used as directed.

- Like over-the-counter remedies, these medicines should only be taken short term. If they have not brought you any significant lasting relief after a few days, you should re-consult your physician.

- A number of herbal and other remedies are available for treating low back pain. These include herbal medicines prescribed by practitioners of traditional Chinese medicine and packaged natural and synthetic compounds sold by health food stores. Herbal medicine has great potential health benefits. The problem with herbal remedies, however, is that their benefits and drawbacks, if any, have not yet been tested in controlled studies. Some of them contain substances that could cause serious harm. For example, many Chinese herbs contain atropine, a substance that affects heart function. Equally important, the quality of herbal remedies varies widely. You cannot always be confident that you are getting the advertised ingredients in the right form. It is far safer to stick with well-tested over-the-counter and prescription medicines.

- Take modified bed rest for two to three days. This means that you should:
  - Spend most of the day resting quietly in the most comfortable position you can find. The two positions that work best for most people are on the side in a slightly fetal position with a pillow between the knees, or flat on the back with the legs raised. The second position really encourages the lower back muscles to relax because it takes all the strain of gravity off them. These are also generally the best positions for sleeping at night.
  - During the day, get up every hour or couple of hours to walk around a little and arch your back backward, to prime the body for a gradual return to full activity. You can also try some light stretching, by pulling each knee up to your chest for a moment or two. Go just to the point where you feel the strain about to become intense, stop there, and take two or three slow, controlled breaths. This is also a good idea if you find you can't sleep through the whole night, which is often the case when a low back injury is fresh.
  - Avoid chair-sitting.
  - Avoid lifting anything heavy.
  - Instead of walking and stretching in the initial recovery phase, seniors should substitute riding a stationary bicycle. Seniors may also find chair-sitting comfortable, because their low back pain usually comes from stenosis, or narrowing of the spine, rather than from a strained muscle or herniated disc. See Chapter 2 for more on these age-related differences.
  - If you have access to a pool, aquatherapy can speed your recovery. Your buoyancy in the water will take all the pressure off the low back.
- In the first twenty-four to forty-eight hours after a low back injury, apply ice to tender areas two to three times a day for ten to fifteen minutes at a time, in order to lessen inflammation. Keeping the ice on for longer won't give you any added benefit; it reaches its maximum efficacy after about ten minutes.
- After twenty-four hours apply moist heat in the shower or with a heating pad for up to thirty minutes at a time as desired. Unlike cold, gentle warmth may continue to provide an increased benefit if it is applied for a longer period of time.
- After twenty-four to forty-eight hours, use heat and ice in sequence. As a general rule, apply heat in the morning and before physical therapy or other

activity; apply ice after activity and in the evening at dinnertime or bedtime. But some people get more relief from heat, whereas others get more from ice, so modify the sequence to fit your own needs.

- Apply liniments and rubs like Tiger Balm, Sportscreme, and BENGAY to soothe injured areas. The "active" ingredients in such products are usually some form of rubbing alcohol, and they never penetrate below skin level. But the act of applying the rub, or having a partner or relative do so for you, can itself be calming and beneficial from an emotional and psycho-physiological point of view.

- As the pain of your injury decreases, gradually increase your activity following the guidelines in Chapter 6 and begin Back Rx Series A.

PART ONE

CHAPTER ONE

HOW YOUR BACK WORKS

THE HEALTHY BACK IS A BACK IN BALANCE

The human back is a marvelously evolved structure, the supportive center of every imaginable movement. We can see that in the way young children roll and tumble as they play, and in the way champion athletes and master practitioners of yoga, Pilates, tai chi, dance, and other movement disciplines have trained their bodies to perform.

The free and easy movement of childhood is everyone's birthright, but most of us have lost it by the time we are adults. That doesn't have to happen. And if we do lose the joy of movement, we can almost always regain it.

One of the most important things to know about the low back is that a high level of pain does not necessarily indicate severe damage. The pain of a low back injury can be worse than a root canal without an anesthetic, but even the most painful injuries seldom pose any serious threat to the spine or brain. The vital parts of the body are simply too well protected for that, except in the most extreme cases. So don't lose hope or fear the worst because the pain is bad. If you follow the pain-relief guidelines on pages xvii–xx and do the exercises in this book for fifteen minutes, three times a week, the odds of a full and lasting recovery are overwhelmingly in your favor.

The human back is so robust because of the way its intricately interwoven parts reinforce each other. The back's function is to support balanced movement and posture and to protect the nerve bundles within the spinal cord. These nerves, the body's information superhighway, carry electrical impulses to and from the brain, where the impulses are translated into sensations, images, emotions, and thoughts.

The back does its job with a hardy structure of bones, muscles, tendons, and ligaments. Layers of muscle—thirty-one muscles tie into the pelvis alone—wrap protectively around the spine, which makes a gentle S-curve from the neck to the tailbone, or coccyx. The spine has twenty-four vertebrae separated and cushioned by the intervertebral discs, which are shock absorbing, doughnut-shaped pads made up of a soft inner portion, the nucleus pulposus, and a hard outer portion, the annulus.

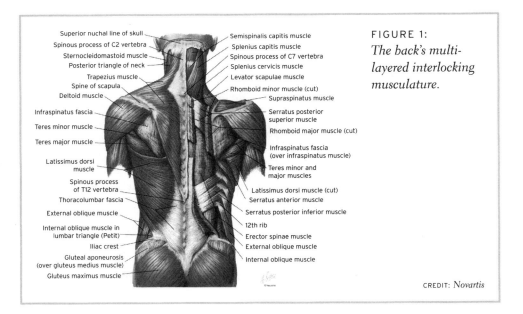

Superior nuchal line of skull
Spinous process of C2 vertebra
Sternocleidomastoid muscle
Posterior triangle of neck
Trapezius muscle
Spine of scapula
Deltoid muscle

Infraspinatus fascia

Teres minor muscle

Teres major muscle

Latissimus dorsi muscle

Spinous process of T12 vertebra
Thoracolumbar fascia

External oblique muscle

Internal oblique muscle in lumbar triangle (Petit)
Iliac crest
Gluteal aponeurosis (over gluteus medius muscle)
Gluteus maximus muscle

Semispinalis capitis muscle
Splenius capitis muscle
Spinous process of C7 vertebra
Splenius cervicis muscle
Levator scapulae muscle
Rhomboid minor muscle (cut)
Supraspinatus muscle

Serratus posterior superior muscle
Rhomboid major muscle (cut)

Infraspinatus fascia (over infraspinatus muscle)
Teres minor and major muscles

Latissimus dorsi muscle (cut)
Serratus anterior muscle
Serratus posterior inferior muscle

12th rib
Erector spinae muscle
External oblique muscle
Internal oblique muscle

FIGURE 1:
The back's multi-layered interlocking musculature.

CREDIT: *Novartis*

4

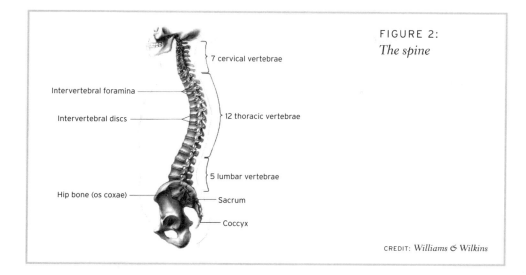

FIGURE 2:
The spine

7 cervical vertebrae

Intervertebral foramina

Intervertebral discs

12 thoracic vertebrae

5 lumbar vertebrae

Hip bone (os coxae)

Sacrum

Coccyx

CREDIT: *Williams & Wilkins*

There are seven cervical, or neck, vertebrae (commonly referred to as C1-C7, counting from top to bottom); twelve thoracic, or chest vertebrae (T1-T12); and five lumbar, or lower back, vertebrae (L1-L5). If a physician or other caregiver diagnoses a low back problem located at disc levels L4-L5, for example, this means that the focal point of the injury is in the area of the fourth and fifth lumbar vertebrae and the disc sandwiched between them.

All of the vertebrae have small projections called facet joints that stabilize the spine and allow it to move in different planes.

Below the fifth lumbar vertebra is the sacrum, a triangular-shaped bone with five segments (S1-S5) that attach to the pelvis (or ilium) to form the sacroiliac joints.

Together with the body's core muscles, the back's S-curve can gently dissipate the energy of harsh impacts or sudden, wrenching movements like a giant spring, and the fluid that fills the soft inner portion of the discs can absorb shocks better than any other known substance. That is, as long as we maintain them in good shape.

At birth the discs are 80% water. As we age, they gradually lose water, stiffen, and turn brittle. Nothing can entirely stop this natural aging process. But as I'll explain in Chapter 4, proper back exercises can be a great age-fighter, dramatically retarding the discs' loss of water and keeping us flexible and resilient.

To stay out of pain, the back has to stay in balance. All of its interlocking parts have to work in harmony. For example, the neuromuscular system works through paired muscles and muscle groups, like the biceps and triceps. The biceps lets you bend your arm, the triceps lets you extend it. Similarly, in the low back, the abdominals let you bend forward, whereas the paraspinal muscles let you extend straight and arch backward. If one muscle or muscle group is disproportionately stronger or weaker than its opposite number, the whole system will suffer.

As I mentioned in the introduction, one muscle imbalance that tends to be especially significant for low back pain is the poor flexion and reduced range of motion in the hips, which results from too much sitting in chairs. In Chapter 2, we'll look more closely at how chair-sitting upsets the body's natural balances and how we can restore them.

The back's need for balance includes a balance of the body and the mind. In terms of the neuromuscular system, a relaxed, balanced posture depends on a host of tiny cells, called proprioceptors, that feed data on position and movement from the muscles, tendons, joints, and inner ear to the brain. To test how proprioception works, try this experiment: Stand on one leg with your arms extended straight out to the sides at shoulder height. You'll probably notice a little wobble, but nothing you can't control. Now increase the difficulty by closing your eyes. The wobble gets worse and before long you'll have to open your eyes and put your foot down to regain your balance. Proprioception is what enables you to hold the position even briefly, and the better your proprioception the longer you'll be able to hold it.

Proprioception underlies all of our body awareness. With good proprioception, we sense intuitively when our bodies are in proper alignment and we instinctively walk and move with good posture and balance. This helps the back by enabling the discs to breathe. Like the rest of the body, the discs depend on the circulatory system to bring them essential, nourishing oxygen. Blood vessels at their periphery are the final stage of this delivery system, so far as the discs are concerned.

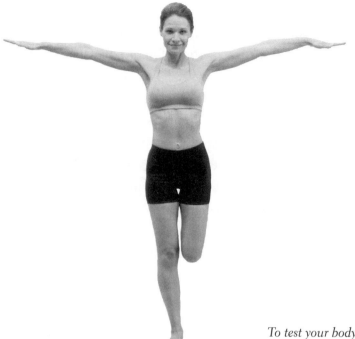

To test your body awareness,
try balancing on one leg.

Walking in balanced alignment with good posture pumps a steady, ample flow of oxygen to the discs with the rhythmic muscular contraction and expansion of every step. By contrast, our modern chair-bound lifestyles cramp the discs into a stressed position and starve them of oxygen for hours at a stretch. This not only weakens abdominal and back muscles and reduces hip flexion and range of motion, it also inevitably degrades our proprioception and body awareness. With this degraded proprioception—a condition that being overweight, out of shape, or a smoker can worsen—we walk and sit hunched over, straining our discs and back muscles with every movement without realizing it. As proprioception weakens, our brains lose the all-important ability to "see" ourselves accurately in space.

The mind's role in low back pain naturally extends to other levels of awareness. Stressful life experiences that agitate our minds and burden us with excessive anxiety, guilt, and other difficult feelings have long been known to be linked with low back pain. And a low back injury can easily trigger a pain-depression cycle that blocks recovery. Over time, an unbalanced state of mind can contribute to low back pain as much as, or more than, any other factor. The bottom line is that if we go too far off-kilter in any area where we need balance—physically, mentally, and/or emotionally—we face an increased risk of low back pain.

All things considered, there is no doubt that balance is the hallmark of a healthy back. When your back is truly in balance, all sorts of tasks become easier to do and life becomes physically, mentally, and emotionally less stressful. Our stress doesn't disappear by any means, but we become energetic and resilient enough to handle it and thrive.

With that in mind, let's look at the mechanisms of low back pain and the specific ways in which the Back Rx program counteracts them, especially the healing power of doing the Back Rx exercises with proper breath control.

CHAPTER TWO

WHY YOUR BACK HURTS

A MIND-BODY PROBLEM

Our backs buckle under a puzzling array of stresses and strains, both major and minor. We can hurt ourselves as easily bending down to tie our shoes as we can digging ditches. A muscle can tighten in extreme pain or a disc can pop as we mow the lawn or bend down to a toddler, as we stoop to pick up a heavy bag or a dropped "Post-it" note, as we exercise and play sports, or as we stand up from sitting in the same position too long. Something as trivial as a sneeze or cough can contort us with low back pain. (In fact, sneezes and coughs subject the torso to very high levels of torque, so here's a tip to reduce the strain: Lean back slightly when you sneeze or cough, instead of bending forward.)

Being in good shape does not guarantee a pain-free back. Elite athletes are as vulnerable to low back injuries as the rest of the population. And just like the rest of us, the world's best athletes can hurt themselves as easily taking out the trash as

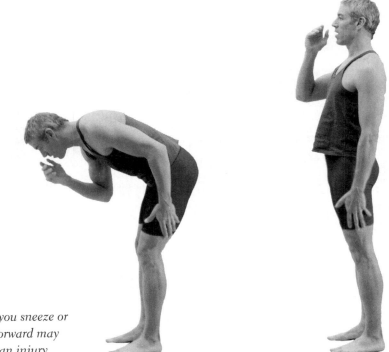

Lean back when you sneeze or cough; bending forward may trigger or worsen an injury.

they can in competition. The sports pages regularly report on athletes who are side-lined by ruptured discs from a variety of causes.

A disc herniates when its soft inner portion, the nucleus pulposus, pushes out through a hole or tear in its tough outer portion, the anulus. Then leaking disc fluid can inflame surrounding tissues, a condition known as chemical radiculitis. If the herniated disc hits a nerve, it can send electric shocks of pain through the back, but-tocks, and legs. Thereafter, because of the body's complex, interconnected struc-ture, the pain can spread to seemingly unrelated areas, such as the neck, shoulders, middle and upper back, abdomen, hips, thighs, and even heels.

Because we felt fine right up until the moment when we turned in an awkward way, lifted a heavy box, sneezed, or bent down to pick up a pencil, we tend to think of that single event as being the one that caused our pain. But far more often than not, the lift or the sneeze is not the ultimate cause of the pain, but only the incident that triggers a painful reaction to accumulated physical, mental, and/or emotional stress and overuse.

If you focus solely on the trigger incident, you risk putting your recovery on a shaky footing. If you look back further, you'll usually recognize that prolonged stress has been making you feel increasingly vulnerable for some time. You'll see, too, that your body has been trying to signal you all along—possibly with subtle symptoms like tightening muscles, increasing tiredness, and minor aches—that you need to slow down and relax a little. But you've been too wound up and distracted by daily obligations and worries to pay attention. Instead of listening to our bodies when injuries are small and can heal quickly, we tend to ignore them until they reach the breaking point.

No doctor can take away your stress. But if you learn how to listen to your body better, you can treat small injuries before they became big ones. You can even avoid injury entirely. In short, the most important treatment you receive for low back pain is not what others give you, but what you give yourself in the form of heightened self-awareness and better self-care.

Good habits of self-care build physical, mental, emotional, and spiritual resilience. In putting self-care front and center, however, I don't mean to suggest that you must heal your back pain all by yourself. Everyone can benefit from others' help in healing. When I hurt my own back, I looked for care and help from others at home and in the doctor's office. In Chapter 3 and Chapter 11 I'll explain how physicians and other caregivers can help you heal your back. But I can't overemphasize that proper self-care—like the Back Rx program—is the foundation for all healing from low back pain.

A LIFESTYLE PROBLEM

One of the things that all of us in the modern world need to pay better attention to is how we punish our backs with chair-sitting. Our backs evolved in a world without furniture to suit a lifestyle of intermittent movement and rest. The best way for our early human ancestors to sit, and surely the most common, was to sit cross-legged flat on the ground.

Much has changed for the better since then, but the healthiest way to sit remains the same. Sitting cross-legged flat on the ground or floor with a straight back engages the whole core body structure—head, neck, shoulders, abdomen, back, and hips—in active harmony. Maintaining a relaxed, balanced posture while sitting cross-legged requires continual micro-adjustments that align the spine, tone muscles and tendons, and perhaps most important, maximize flexion and range of motion in the hips.

Try it for a while, and you'll see. The sooner you feel a telltale strain in your hips, the more vulnerable your back is to injury.

By contrast, sitting in chairs disengages some of these core body elements and puts enormous strain on others. As I mentioned in the introduction, my research indicates that chair-sitting contributes to measurable deficits in hip flexion and range of motion, even in highly conditioned professional athletes. Worst of all, chair-sitting maximizes pressure on the discs and decreases their oxygen supply.

Remember, the discs breathe by taking in oxygen from blood vessels at their periphery. But we suffocate our discs by sitting in chairs too often and for too long. We sit in chairs, in a disc-freezing posture, even when we're "relaxing," while watching television, surfing the Internet, reading, or playing a video game.

It would be a saving grace if we at least walked from one daily activity to another. Instead we sit down in chairs to travel in trains, planes, and automobiles. Most car manufacturers now describe their car seats as ergonomic. Luxury car makers, in particular, like to boast about their body-friendly seats. Unfortunately, even an ergonomic car seat will not significantly reduce disc pressure. The basic chair-sitting posture defeats every ergonomic tweak that the car companies devise.

Back health is much better in the Third World, where many people still grow up sitting cross-legged on the ground or floor and walking from one activity to another, and where relatively few people spend their workdays in a desk chair. In the Third World, backs breathe better.

The final piece of the low back pain puzzle is age-related. In Chapter 1, I mentioned that the discs are 80% water at birth and gradually dry out as we grow older.

During midlife, at least in the developed world, prolonged chair-sitting constitutes a form of overuse that predisposes us to disc bulges and herniations. From about age fifty on, the spinal canal begins to narrow, a condition known as spinal stenosis. Not all stenosis produces problems. But stenosis can cause back pain by putting undue pressure on the nerves that lead out from the sides of the spine. In addition, the increased pressure it puts on the bones of the spine, especially the facet and SI joints, can lead to arthritis. As I'll explain in the next chapter, disc problems and stenosis affect the back differently and require different treatments.

These three Magnetic Resonance Imaging (MRI) scans (Figures 3–5) show the discs at three stages of the life cycle. The first shows a young person's healthy, well-hydrated discs. The second shows a middle-aged person's discs with dehydration under way and a herniation of the disc at L4–L5. In the last, age-related stenosis is beginning to become problematic.

Fortunately, proper exercise that increases the back's flexibility, strength, and endurance, and thus makes good balance and posture possible, can dramatically retard these natural aging processes and moderate their effects.

The bottom line is that low back pain needs a recovery program that will give first aid to injured muscles and discs; tune up poorly developed muscles and tendons in our hips; and help us learn to listen to our bodies to enhance proprioception and

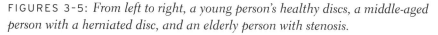
FIGURES 3-5: *From left to right, a young person's healthy discs, a middle-aged person with a herniated disc, and an elderly person with stenosis.*

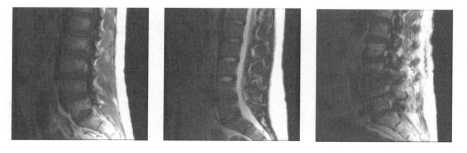

body awareness throughout the life cycle. Back Rx treats both sides of this complicated mind-body puzzle. Its combination of physical therapy exercises with medical adaptations of yoga and Pilates can reset the balance between core muscle groups. At the same time, its calming breath control can reset the balance between the body and the mind.

Now let's look closely at how Back Rx can help you progress successfully through every stage of low back pain care and recovery.

CHAPTER THREE

THE FOUR STAGES OF LOW BACK PAIN CARE AND RECOVERY

Treatments for low back pain fall into four main categories or stages. The vast majority of patients can achieve full recovery with Stage I care. You become a candidate for Stage II care and beyond only if you are among the roughly 20% of low back pain sufferers who do not heal during Stage I. Each additional stage of care is in turn appropriate for a smaller and smaller patient pool.

STAGE I CARE

Stage I care is for just about everyone with low back pain. It involves a sequenced combination of rest, medications (anti-inflammatories, muscle relaxants, and pain relievers as needed), heat and ice, and gentle rehabilitative exercise. Back Rx is a comprehensive program of Stage I care.

This first stage of care can resolve 80% or more of all low back problems. It should not be bypassed or curtailed, unless surgery is indicated as described on page 17. When other treatments are tried, Back Rx or a similar program of Stage I care should almost always be continued, or resumed as soon as possible afterward, in order to realize their full benefits.

Stage I care may be complemented by traditional physical therapy, osteopathy, medical massage, chiropractic, acupuncture, or some combination of these. For more information on these treatments and how to decide if they're right for you, see the rest of this chapter and Chapter 11.

STAGE II CARE

For severe, ongoing low back pain that does not respond to Stage I care, Stage II offers three minimally-invasive, nonsurgical procedures:

- In cases of low back pain without leg pain, paravertebral, or trigger point, injections of a saline solution to inflamed, tender areas.
- Selective nerve root epidurals under fluoroscopy, also known as guided epidurals. These injections deliver a carefully calibrated dose of lidocaine and corticosteroid directly to the inflamed nerve that is the source of the pain, as determined with the aid of fluoroscopy. (Fluoroscopy is a form of X-ray guidance.) These injections are used for low back pain with leg pain (sciatica) and have a high, long-lasting success rate when combined with icing and an exercise regimen like Back Rx.
- Facet and sacroiliac (SI) joint injections are also done under fluoroscopy for pain that is deemed to originate from these deep structures. The drawback of these injections is that their effect may be temporary, even if combined with icing and proper exercise.

STAGE III CARE

For low back pain that does not respond to Stage II care, Stage III care offers three nonsurgical, and two surgical, procedures:

- Radio Frequency Denervation, which halts pain in the facet and SI joints by heating the nerves, which innervates these joints, making the nerves inactive for a couple of years. The procedure can then be repeated.
- Intradiscal Electrothermal Therapy (IDET), which heats the annulus, the hard outer portion of an injured disc.
- Nucleoplasty, which heats the nucleus pulposus, the softer inner portion of an injured disc.
- Micro-discectomy and laminectomy, two very similar surgical procedures in which the herniated portion of a disc is removed.

STAGE IV CARE

Stage IV care options remain limited, for the present, to spinal fusions, which can be effective in cases of combined back and leg pain. But within the next two to three years artificial disc replacement, which is now being studied in U.S. Food and Drug Administration (FDA) trials, should become widely available.

For more information on Stage II to Stage IV care options, and which ones may be appropriate for you, see Chapter 12. For now, keep in mind that well over 95% of all low back pain cases can be healed without surgery. Surgery is indicated only

- To stop the progressive loss of neurological function
- To restore bowel and bladder function
- To end intractable pain.

If you've hurt your back and find that you're losing an increasing amount of feeling and sensation in the leg or elsewhere in the body, that you can't go to the bathroom (this is no joke, but a potentially life-threatening problem), or that severe pain persists no matter what you do, you should put down this book and seek an evaluation from a qualified physician as soon as possible.

The potential for such complications is frightening, and in the immediate aftermath of back injury or reinjury, when the pain is overwhelming, it can be hard not to fear the worst. But once again, please remember that almost all low back pain sufferers can achieve a full and lasting recovery with a sound program of Stage I care like Back Rx, especially if they have the right caregivers in their corner.

A PHYSICIAN'S HELP

You can do Back Rx or a similar program entirely on your own. But a physician's expert guidance can help keep your recovery on track and progressing optimally. Primary care physicians are well equipped to manage low back pain, coordinate the efforts of specialist physicians, physical therapists, and other caregivers, and coach you through your recovery. During Stage I care, they can provide the insight and support you need to stick with Back Rx or a similar program long enough for full healing to occur.

The specialist physicians most often involved in low back care are physiatrists, neurologists, anesthesiologists, orthopedic surgeons, and neurosurgeons. Except for physiatrists, specialist M.D.s do not participate much in Stage I care. In later stages of care, a neurologist can be helpful if a person is suffering from foot drop or other signs of neurological weakness. If it becomes necessary to explore surgical interventions such as a discectomy, orthopedic surgeons and neurosurgeons with fellowship training in spinal surgery have state-of-the-art spinal surgical skills. They also have the expertise to offer informed second opinions on prospective surgery. In cases of ongoing severe pain, especially pain that persists after surgery, anesthesiologists with pain management fellowship training should be consulted.

The first consultations with specialist physicians should occur within six months of injury, if possible. After six months, healing becomes a lot harder and the prognosis for full recovery from a low back problem becomes less favorable.

As primary care physicians for the musculoskeletal system and specialists in physical medicine and rehabilitation, physiatrists can play a healing role at every stage of low back care. All physiatrists receive extensive training in conservative nonsurgical care for the low back. Additional subspecialty training in physiatry, such as a fellowship in spine and sports medicine, can be particularly useful in later treatment stages, because it provides expertise in minimally invasive, nonsurgical spinal treatments combined with proper rehabilitation.

All things considered, in the event of a low back problem you should probably turn first to your present primary care physician and his or her referral network. Someone who knows you and your medical history, and whom you trust and feel comfortable with, has a better chance of getting your recovery in high gear quickly and managing it smoothly than a doctor who is meeting you for the first time.

If you do need to find a doctor from scratch, whether a general practitioner or a specialist, the best way to find any good caregiver is through word-of-mouth recommendations from people you trust. You can also learn about different medical specialties and find referrals on the websites of physicians' groups. At the end of the book you'll find an appendix with a list of organizations and websites that can help you with your search.

OTHER CAREGIVERS

In addition to general practice and specialist M.D.s, a number of other caregivers treat low back pain, including physical therapists, osteopaths, massage therapists, chiropractors, and acupuncturists. Whereas M.D.s and physical therapists are said to practice conventional medicine, the other caregivers are often said to practice integrated medicine. I find these labels a little awkward. Every good healer wants to take an integrated, holistic approach to patient care. "Leave no stone unturned to help the patient" should be every caregiver's motto.

Granted that, and granted that equally good healers can have very different credentials, you want to make sure that the caregivers you go to have the appropriate credentials for their different fields. Keep in mind that whereas conventional medicine regularly tests its practices in controlled studies, most of integrated medicine has not yet been documented with the same rigor. Of the common alternatives to conventional medical care for the low back, only massage therapy and osteopathy have so far been proven effective in clinical trials. There is other, if less rigorous, medical evidence for the value of acupuncture and chiropractic, however, and I have seen many patients helped by each of them.

To find a good practitioner of one of these treatments, ask around. Personal recommendations from people you know and trust are the best way to find a good healer. After that you have to follow your instincts. Everyone is different, and every case of low back pain is different. As long as you are making an informed choice, you should feel free to pick and choose the therapies that seem best suited to your individual needs, perspective, and lifestyle. The proof is then in the pudding. A therapy may be very appealing for one reason or another, and it may help other people. But if it doesn't help you over the course of a few weeks or months, you should abandon it and move on to something else. As with conventional medical care, you should try to find the right integrated medical care for your case within six months of your injury. After that point, healing becomes much harder, no matter what the treatment is.

I'll have more to say about these varied treatment options in Chapter 11. Here I would only caution that where chiropractic is concerned, you should not have any high-velocity manipulations of the head and neck. They can cause spinal cord injuries and strokes. It's not a high risk, but why take the chance that you'll be the one person in many thousands who is crippled or killed?

SELF-CARE MAKES ALL THE DIFFERENCE

I've already emphasized the importance of self-care in treating low back pain. Good habits of self-care build physical, mental, emotional, and spiritual resilience. When it comes to receiving low back treatments from others, the enhanced body awareness that develops from effective self-care will help you to choose the treatments that are best suited to your own case and to get the most out of those treatments.

The array of potential treatments for low back pain is enormous. Conventional medicine, osteopathy, physical therapy, massage, acupuncture, and chiropractic can all benefit people with low back injuries, but in my experience, some are more effective at one stage of recovery than another. And at every stage of recovery, some of these things work better for some people than they do for others. Moreover, none of them can guarantee a cure. Good self-care can make all the difference, enabling you to leverage the power of the treatments you receive from others. Professional athletes can often heal astonishingly quickly, simply because of how well they have learned to listen to their bodies and how they are able to use their body knowledge to guide those who care for them.

At the core of what Back Rx teaches are habits of self-care and self-attunement that can ultimately transform your relationship with your body. Most of all, Back Rx trains you to tune clearly and surely into the stream of signals that the body is always processing. When you make a habit of listening to these signals on a regular basis, they tell you which muscles need stretching and strengthening and what the limit of the effort should be. They guide you to apply the gradually increasing, moderate stresses that aid healing, and to avoid the extreme stresses that retard it. The body's proprioceptive faculties also "tell" you more and more accurately when you are in proper alignment and balance for any activity and when you're not, helping you to maintain the good posture and flowing movement that ultimately keep back injuries from occurring.

As you build a habit of listening to your body while you do the Back Rx exercises, you develop the ability to "listen" more and more at a subliminal level throughout the day, without the need for conscious attention. Eventually you'll reach the point where you notice right away when stress and overuse are beginning to affect your back, and you'll then be able to take proactive steps to moderate and even prevent episodes of low back pain before they occur. Ultimately you'll become able to direct this sharpened mental focus and enhanced energy to boost your performance in every area of your life.

One of the best ways to help further this process, after the initial inflammation and severe pain of an acute injury have subsided, is through self-massage and partner massage. All healing needs the human touch, and none more so than low back pain. The first thing to realize about self-massage is that you can't hurt yourself. At most, if you really got carried away, you might give yourself a superficial bruise, but you can't exert enough pressure with your own unaided hands to damage anything below the skin level.

But if you can't apply enough pressure to hurt yourself more than a little bit, you can easily apply enough pressure to help yourself a lot. You can massage and manipulate your own body to a remarkable degree, if you do so with a sense of play and a willingness to experiment.

The way to start is to put your fingers or hands on the injured areas and rest them there for a moment. You're about to get reacquainted with your body—you've probably been injured so badly in the first place because you've literally lost proprioceptive touch with your body—and there's no need to rush.

Now focus on your breathing. Slow it down. Exhale fully. Empty your lungs. Inhale slowly and deeply. Hold the breath for a count of three. Exhale slowly and continue the cycle for ten breaths.

As you rest your hands or fingers on the injured areas of your body and breathe in this slow, controlled, sustained way, your body will begin to tell you how it wants to be touched, rubbed, kneaded, pressed, and prodded into alignment. The knots in the muscle tissue that are keeping your body from relaxing into its natural alignment are bunched up around, and are themselves largely composed of, small sacs of water. As Rick Sharpel, a leading medical massage therapist in New York, puts it, "Massage works by moving those tiny sacs of water so that they spread out smoothly along the entire length of the muscle, rather than being bunched up in the belly of the muscle."

Medical massage generally treats the belly of tight muscles by rubbing crossways—called cross-fiber massage—more than lengthwise. You can use any part of the fingers, knuckles, hands, wrists, or forearms to do this. A massage therapist or a gentle, trusted partner might also use the elbows to apply sufficient steady pressure to reach and unkink severe muscle strains.

You can even use objects to do massage. There are many household objects you can use, from a solid doorjamb to a bag full of tennis or golf balls. Put a towel over the bag of golf balls or other object—some people even like to use a rock with a definite edge or point—and then carefully lie down on the floor on your back. Rest your lower back on the object and begin to apply the pressure where and how your body says it helps. If you are doing some rehabilitation work at a gym or under the supervision of a therapist, you might also use an extra-large-diameter sports ball to lie back and roll around on.

The amount of pressure that you apply or a massage therapist applies is obviously a critical factor. As a general rule, the more relaxed you are, the more that steadily increasing pressure will be pleasurable rather than painful. But when massage therapy reaches the point of maximum tenderness—some massage therapists call it the point of exquisite pain—you have to be willing to endure some increased short-term discomfort in the interest of better healing. This healthy stress is produced by slow, sustained, controlled movements and gradual increases in pressure to a point just below your pain threshold, not by sharp, stabbing actions or sharp, stabbing pain at or above that threshold.

If you keep these simple ideas in mind, you can do wonders for yourself with self-massage. At the very least you'll gain an increased knowledge of your body that most people lack and that can guide your further healing and safeguard you against recurrences.

Here is a self-massage tip to get you started:

Stand up straight with your feet parallel and shoulder distance apart. Let your shoulders hang down your back—don't hunch them up to your neck. Look straight ahead out the window or at an imaginary horizon. Imagine that a string hanging straight down from the sky is attached to the top of your head and is gently pulling your spine straight and lengthening it.

Now rest your hands on your hips. All your body parts are proportional, so in this position your thumbs will be on the lines of the paraspinal muscles that extend up and down on both sides of the spine. Your fingertips will be touching the psoas muscles in your abdomen. From this hand position you can apply soothing pressure front and back and up and down through the zone of your low back injury.

This is an especially good self-massage starter because it works pairs of muscles, front and back. The Back Rx exercises also work paired muscle groups front and back, because it is only their combined operation that enables and supports balance and movement in the first place. For the body's muscles to work in this harmonious way, they must have good flexibility, strength, and endurance. Let's now explore how these three factors combine to keep the back in balance and pain-free.

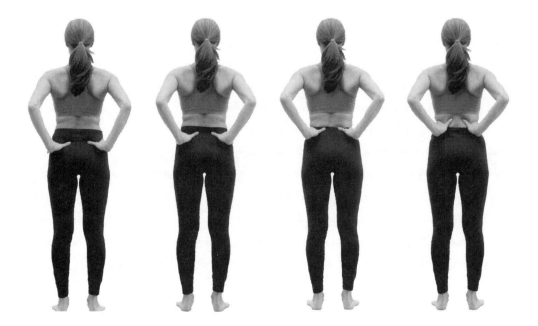

CHAPTER FOUR

FLEXIBILITY, STRENGTH, AND ENDURANCE: THE THREE KEYS TO GOOD BALANCE AND POSTURE

Maintaining an injury-resistant and resilient back, with good balance and posture, depends on three interrelated components of muscle health: flexibility, strength, and endurance.

- **FLEXIBILITY** is the ability to absorb and channel forces within the body, to bend without breaking.
- **STRENGTH** is the ability to exert force.
- **ENDURANCE** is the ability to do these things again and again without tiring.

All of these three factors are involved in every move we make. Flexibility forms the essential foundation for strength and endurance, and a lack of flexibility carries an increased risk of injury during training for strength and endurance.

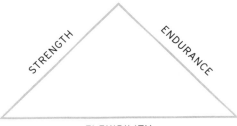

STRENGTH   ENDURANCE

FLEXIBILITY

FLEXIBILITY TO BEND WITHOUT BREAKING

Flexibility is vitally important to muscle health. The muscles in our bodies form part of a neuromuscular system, a vast network of pathways for the flow of electrical energy in the form of nerve signals and impulses. In order for muscles to come into action smoothly and efficiently, these signals need to flow through our muscle fibers and other tissues like water coursing through a mountain stream. There should be no stiffness blocking these signals.

The fluid flow of nerve impulses through the body is what enables elite athletes to generate explosive power, just as a supple flick of the wrist can send a tidal wave of energy crackling through a whip. Professional golfers' swings illustrate the importance of flexibility. Consider John Daly and Tiger Woods, for example. They have vastly different body types, one as couch potatoey as the other is muscular, but both have extreme flexibility. Both golfers twist their bodies like pretzels in order to generate the high clubhead speed that is needed to hit the ball long. The difference is that John Daly's flexibility seems to be almost entirely genetic, whereas Tiger Woods' flexibility is clearly the product of sustained, well-focused training and conditioning.

Injuries tend to occur in the phases of a movement—those involved in preparing to generate or absorb a force—that most depend on flexibility. When part of the neuromuscular system is too stiff or tight, shear forces can easily build to the point where tissues tear and joints get ground together or wrenched apart.

In this regard, flexibility often turns out to be a question of muscle relationships as well as individual muscles. My colleague Robert Donatelli, Ph.D., P.T., of Atlanta, Georgia, one of the country's foremost physical therapists, was consulted by a major league baseball player who had suffered repeated hamstring injuries. Long known as a gifted all-around player with a lethal bat, this major leaguer could no longer hit with power or sprint between the bases. He couldn't even sit down for longer than twenty minutes without intense low back and leg pain. Many coaches, trainers, and strength experts had tried to fix the problem without success, all by focusing more or less entirely on the hamstrings. Bob Donatelli took a different approach, focusing on the muscles in the inner trunk, the multifidis and abdominal muscles, that should ideally work in fluid concert with the hamstrings. When the strength of these inner trunk muscles was raised to balance the strength of the leg muscles, the player's hamstring tightness disappeared, his pain stopped, and he quickly recaptured his peak performance abilities, extending his major league career after a number of baseball and fitness experts had written him off. I have seen similar things happen with many professional golfers and tennis players.

Most of us will never compete at the high level of professional athletes. But as Bob Donatelli puts it, "Elite athletes are like laboratory subjects for the rest of us. They're out there every day testing the limits of the human system." We can learn from them, because the explosive movements of competitive sports are really very close to the explosive stresses that we all encounter, for example, when we slip and try to stop ourselves from falling, when we stand up or bend down abruptly after being locked into position at our desks for hours at a stretch, or when we're playing recreational sports or working out as weekend warriors.

Flexibility means different things for different kinds of muscles. Some muscles in the body are stabilizers; they hold bones in place. Other muscles are mobilizers; they move bones in space. These two types of muscle are made up of different kinds of muscle fibers. Stabilizing muscles, like the core inner muscles of the trunk, the multifidis and the abdominals, contain a preponderance of Type I fibers, which fire isometrically and hold contractions in one place. Mobilizing muscles, like the biceps, contain a preponderance of Type II fibers, which fire through dynamic expansion and contraction. You can tell the difference immediately if you clench your abs, then lift something with one arm.

As the Type I fibers in the core trunk muscles contract, they stiffen the spinal area to absorb the shock of generating a whip-action movement like a golf swing, a tennis serve, or an abrupt stoop down to pick up a pencil. Even more important, they stiffen the spinal area in order to handle the stress of decelerating that movement without injury.

This response can be trained, and the core muscles can be developed to accommodate greater forces, just as the dynamic muscle strength of the biceps can be trained to lift more and more weight. A study in Italy found that training core flexibility dramatically reduced injuries among soccer-playing kids. One group of children trained according to conventional methods, while the other did exercises that focused on bringing the inner trunk muscles into action more smoothly and rapidly. In the year after their training, the first group experienced twice as many ligament tears as the second group.

FLEXIBILITY, THE AGE-FIGHTER

There's one more aspect of flexibility to consider as you seek relief from low back pain, and that is its connection to the life cycle. The older we get the less flexible we become, because our tissues lose water and dry out as part of aging. The loss of water from our tissues begins as a very gradual process, but it picks up momentum in midlife. In people who smoke or who are overweight, the process speeds up even sooner. When the loss of water in tissues becomes severe, the discs and other parts of the body actually shrink and collapse in on themselves. This is what bends some elderly people into a C-shape with a crooked back. On an MRI, as we saw in Chapter 2, discs with good water content appear light colored or white, and dehydrated discs appear dark.

Nothing can reverse this process. Stopping smoking, losing weight, and drinking plenty of fluids will all help slow it down (drink ¼ ounce of water per pound of body weight a day in cool weather, and ½ ounce in hot weather). But flexibility training can retard it dramatically. Lifelong yogists, for example, frequently retain well-hydrated discs into advanced old age. Paradoxically, this means that they can herniate discs even in their sixties or later, when most people's discs are well on the way to becoming dried-out husks. One of my patients, Simon B., herniated a disc at age sixty-eight. When we looked at his MRIs, he had the white, well-hydrated discs of a young man, thanks to forty years of involvement with yoga. Although he needed Back Rx medical yoga during his recovery phase before he could return to his normal yoga routines, those routines had kept his back in remarkably good shape. My own grandfather Gangadhar is also a case in point. Through daily yoga practice he remained supple and erect until his death at the age of ninety-one. At eighty-five he took a trip around the world, and he had a spring in his step and a glint in his eye at every stop along the way.

Flexibility training can pay off even if you begin it late in life. Another patient of mine was a fifty-six-year-old racquetball player who had never done any flexibility work. When he came to see me, he was suffering from recurring episodes of debilitating right-side low back pain. I prescribed ice, anti-inflammatories, and Back Rx. He committed himself to doing the Back Rx exercises daily, and eight months later he was both pain-free and much more flexible. His enhanced flexibility will help protect against further injury to his low back, and it will also retard the aging of his entire body.

The sooner you begin a gradual program of flexibility training and the longer you continue it, the healthier your discs will be and the more you can retard your own aging process.

STRENGTH TO MOVE

Researchers in biomechanics define strength as the body's ability to produce force through the contraction and expansion of muscles. More specifically, they separate muscle action into four categories:

1. Isometric, in which a muscle contracts in place but does not lengthen. Clenching your abdominals is an example of isometric contraction.
2. Concentric, in which a muscle contracts and shortens, as when the biceps contracts and shortens in lifting a dumbbell.
3. Eccentric, in which a muscle lengthens. The biceps lengthens, but remains in tension, as the arm straightens in lowering a dumbbell.
4. Plyometric, in which concentric and eccentric contractions alternate. This is a question both of individual muscles and of paired muscle groups. Just as the biceps contracts and lengthens as a dumbbell is raised and lowered, the triceps does the opposite, lengthening as the biceps contracts and contracting as the biceps lengthens.

Another important way of distinguishing these different kinds of muscle action is that isometric contractions are static and do not involve movement, whereas concentric, eccentric, and plyometric contractions are dynamic and involve moving the body, or a part of the body, in space.

Most body movements, like bending down to pick something up from the floor and standing up again, involve a series of linked isometric and plyometric contractions. No muscle in the body works in isolation. Both individual muscles and muscle groups work together in pairs.

Muscle strength is not primarily a question of muscle size. A large, healthy muscle will, of course, be stronger than a small one. But far more important is how fluidly and efficiently the nervous system can recruit both individual muscles and paired muscle groups to produce muscular force. Full recruitment of a "weak" muscle can produce more force than partial recruitment of a "strong" one.

Back health requires not only that individual muscles in the trunk, hips, and thighs be strong, but also that core muscle groups work together properly. Thirty-one muscles tie into the pelvis, for example, and they all need to act in harmony. The stronger the trunk muscles are, and the more balanced they are in strength, the less pressure there will be on the spine's intervertebral discs and facet joints and the more resistant a person will be to disc herniations, facet arthritis, and other back problems.

ENDURANCE TO WITHSTAND STRESS

Life is a marathon, and we all need endurance to stay in the race. Luckily, we can train for neuromuscular endurance, increasing our energy reserves so that we never run out of gas. A high level of endurance enables the body to bounce back supple and erect after a strenuous ordeal, whether that ordeal is a twenty-six-mile run or another typical day of juggling family, work, and relationship stress.

Competitive athletes devote a lot of time to endurance training. A professional tennis player with a booming 125-mph serve must be able to repeat that serve without tiring all the way through a five-set match. Sure, top competitors do get tired in hard-fought contests. They may be physically and emotionally drained at the end, but if they have achieved a sufficient level of endurance, they will not have fatigued their bodies to the point of injury or beyond.

Most people don't tax their core muscles with explosive physical forces over and over again, the way competitive athletes do. But the prolonged stresses of normal living can be equally hard on the back, especially given the well-documented role of emotional factors in low back injuries and chronic pain. And unlike professional athletes, most of us can't devote full time to recovering from an injury, and we don't have elaborate support systems of nutritionists, trainers, and therapists to help us heal. Our lives just don't stop and wait for us when we get sick. Endurance training can play a big role in preventing injuries and in shortening recovery times if we do get injured.

THE RIGHT AMOUNT OF ENDURANCE WORK FOR YOU

Although everyone can benefit from appropriate endurance training, the right training for an elite athlete and a working mother probably won't be the same (unless the working mother is an elite athlete). Depending on your fitness level and lifestyle, Back Rx Series A, B, or C can provide all the endurance training you need. Over time, the slow, steady, moderate stresses and focused breathing of each series can build very healthy levels of endurance along with core strength. See Part 2 for guidelines on which series is right for you as your recovery progresses.

Guided imagery can enhance this process enormously. For example, if you imagine that a warm golden light is filling your body, focusing on that image can help you to control your breathing better and thus hold the proper posture longer, which in turn builds endurance. Or you might imagine yourself doing the exercises in some favorite place where you feel secure and at ease emotionally, like a forest glade or a pristine beach. In addition to making your back feel better, guiding workouts with your own positive images will heighten your powers of concentration, which can add clarity and creativity to problem solving of all kinds. Choosing your own images also builds confidence, and that, too, makes you better able to meet all sorts of challenges successfully.

BALANCE BRINGS EASE

An appropriate mix of flexibility, strength, and endurance training, like that in Back Rx, will put you well on the way to building a strong, healthy back. To reach that goal, and maintain it with consistent good balance and posture, however, requires putting the mind and proper breathing at the center of everything.

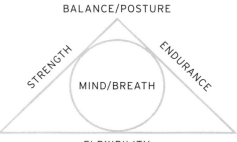

As we have seen, there are two interconnected reasons for this. First, the well-documented link between psychological and emotional stress and low back problems gives mind-calming breath control an important role to play in healing these ailments and preventing their recurrence.

Second, persistent or recurrent physical and emotional problems, such as low back pain, disrupt the mind-body connection, contributing to a loss of proprioception, the faculty that gives us a sense of body position even with our eyes closed.

Doing Back Rx consistently can greatly enhance your mental and physical balance. You not only become better able to bend without breaking physically, but you also grow more in tune with yourself mentally. You are thus better able to defuse stressful situations and reduce both physical and emotional tension before it accumulates to the danger point.

If you are angry, anxious, depressed, or frightened, using Back Rx's focused breathing techniques to calm yourself can save you from sliding into a negative downward spiral. The ability to step back from feelings of frustration and upset can also save you from saying and doing things in the heat of the moment that you wish you hadn't. That can be a lifesaver in all sorts of situations, whether at home, work, or play. Losing your temper on the tennis court or golf course, for example, is often the prelude to a breakdown in technique and focus that invites injury. In contrast, learning to reconnect with a calm mental center puts you back in control of yourself, so that stress no longer calls the shots.

This is why Back Rx puts mind at the center of recovery and healing. The payoff for doing so can be profound and can manifest itself on many levels, because a balance of mind and body brings ease. There is really no limit to the extent to which you can use Back Rx to tune up your mental and physical functioning, because it helps you learn to listen to your body better and heed its warning signals sooner rather than later.

The ultimate payoff of Back Rx is that it gradually enhances your mind and body awareness so that your posture is well balanced and the mind-body system can operate optimally. Posture is the visible expression not just of a physical state, but of the relationship between mind and body. Hunched, bent-forward postures maximize disc pressures and indicate that this relationship is out of balance. Supple, erect posture minimizes disc pressures and indicates a true inner harmony of mind and body that will stand us in good stead no matter how we have to bend and twist to meet life's challenges.

If you commit yourself to the habits of good self-care in the Back Rx program, you will see how a relaxed body can translate into a calming clarity of mind. Then the mere act of standing tall and taking deep, gentle breaths can re-energize you and help you solve problems in all areas of your life.

CHAPTER FIVE

POWER TIPS FOR HEALTHY BACKS

Regular Back Rx workouts will put your back in shape to respond easily and intuitively to almost any challenge that life brings your way. In addition, here are some practical tips I often give my patients.

SLEEPING

The best sleeping position for you is the one you find most comfortable and restful. In general, sleeping on your side with your knees slightly bent puts the least pressure on the spinal discs and low back. Putting a small pillow between your knees will decrease the pressure even more.

If you prefer to sleep on your back, try using a bolster or some firm pillows to elevate your lower legs. This will flatten out the low back and decrease the pressure on the discs.

A medium-firm mattress, which can either be a conventional mattress or a futon, is best. It should be well supported on a solid bed-frame, a box spring, or even the floor.

Some manufacturers make rather bold claims for their mattresses' ability to help your back. You can spend many thousands of dollars on one of these mattresses, and probably get quite a good mattress. But there's certainly no medical evidence to show that an extremely expensive mattress is better for your back than a more reasonably priced one.

SEX

While recovering from a back injury, men and women alike should let their partners be the more active, athletic ones. It is best to lie on your back or side until you're really feeling like yourself again. In the meantime, you can let a gentle, loving touch be part of your recovery in any way you find comfortable.

SHOES AND ORTHOTICS

The feet are vitally important to good back health. As the first link in a kinetic muscle chain that extends upward to the knees, hips, and back, the feet must be flexible enough to adapt to uneven surfaces and absorb shock, but they must also lock into a rigid position to push off from the ground or floor. If there is a biomechanical deficiency or misalignment in the feet, excessive force can be transmitted up the muscle chain to cause or worsen low back pain.

Everyone's feet spread out over the course of the day, so make sure your shoes are roomy enough to allow for this. Studies have shown that the majority of women, almost 90%, hurt their health by wearing shoes that are too small for them, and men often make the same mistake. To help your feet be better shock absorbers, your shoes should also provide good heel and arch support and have a rigid or semirigid sole. Properly fitted running and fitness walking shoes provide this combination of features.

Obviously there are some occasions in life when style rules, but insofar as possible, all your shoes should fit like your most comfortable running shoes.

Negative-slope shoes, which keep the toes higher than the heels, are sometimes touted as being back-friendly. But before buying a pair, you may want to consider the fact that this is a serious distortion of the body's natural biomechanics. Over time, this can distort muscle balances in the foot and lower leg.

A medical examination for low back pain should always include the feet and ankles. If there is a misalignment or other problem in these areas, such as fallen or overly high arches, orthotic shoe inserts can often help. But as Dr. Rock Positano, my colleague at the Hospital for Special Surgery and co-director of the Foot Center at New York Presbyterian Hospital/Weill-Cornell Medical Center, cautions, orthotics are definitely a prescription item that require expert diagnosis and fitting. Inserts you buy over the counter or on the Internet can easily worsen the problem you are trying to correct.

BACK BRACES

A supportive back brace can be helpful in the first two to three weeks of recovery from an acute episode of low back pain, especially if it has a pocket to hold an ice bag or heat pack. If you wear a brace for too long, however, your core muscles—the very ones that must become stronger to heal your pain long term—begin to atrophy. So don't rely on a brace for longer than a month without consulting a physician.

DESK AND COMPUTER SETUP

If modern life didn't keep people sitting at desks so much of the time, there would be a great deal less low back pain in the world. Since that situation is not going to change, however, we all need to practice common sense as we work at our computer screens and file-strewn desks.

Let's start with the chair. A number of very expensive ergonomic chairs have come on the market in the last few years, and a couple of them have become high-tech fashion statements. There's nothing wrong with that, but even the best designed and manufactured chair cannot eliminate the effect of gravity. Your own body awareness in the chair is the most important factor affecting your posture in it. The enhanced proprioception that Back Rx develops, for example, can keep you alert to the increasing disc pressure that comes from bending forward over your laptop computer for twenty or thirty minutes at a stretch. That pressure reminds you to practice the healthy back habit of getting out of your chair every twenty or thirty minutes to:

stand tall,
arch backward,
do a little paraspinal thumb massage (see Chapter 3),
and, most of all, breathe fully and deeply for thirty to forty seconds.

This takes the pressure off the discs and lets them breathe. It is the best thing you can do to prevent office work from injuring your back. An ergonomic chair is still a good idea, but you don't have to spend a fortune to get one.

Pick the chair not by how it looks, but by how you feel in it. It should accommodate your body-type well, have a medium-firm cushion or seat, and adjust in height so that your thighs are parallel to the floor when you sit down in it. Built-in lumbar support is a plus, but you can also get that benefit from a fasten-on lumbar support (available at office supply stores).

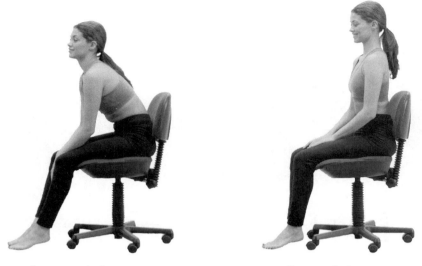

Incorrect chair posture   *Correct chair posture*

Your posture in the chair should be erect, yet supple, with the top of your head, your ears, your shoulders, and your hips aligned, not rigidly, but more or less in the same flexible plane. Your shoulders should not be hunched up or bent forward, as if they were attached to your neck. The shoulders are attached to the back, and they need to hang out easily behind and below your neck. When they do, your shoulders straighten and your neck muscles relax.

Finally, don't jut your jaw out and up when you are sitting or standing. A poor computer setup can encourage this position, which strains your neck and back. It also constricts your breathing. Try instead to relax the back of your neck, making it long and straight so that you can look at the computer screen straight ahead or at a gentle angle down. Your jaw should gently drop down a few fractions of an inch toward your chest, allowing the long cylinder of your windpipe to open easily. In this position you can breathe almost as fully and evenly sitting down in your chair as you can standing up.

The idea is not to try to sit permanently fixed in one alignment, but to establish the position you want your body to keep relaxing into, aided by good proprioception and balance, as well as by core body flexibility, strength, and endurance.

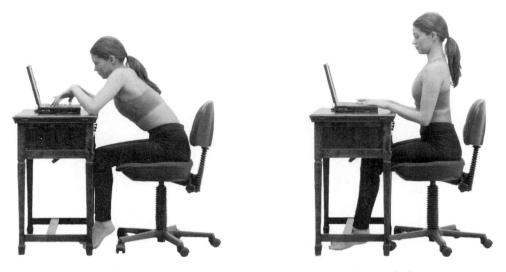

Incorrect desk posture   *Correct desk posture*

The chair's relation to the work surface is also important. As you sit upright in the chair, you should be able to rest your elbows easily on the work surface with your forearms more or less parallel with the floor. When you are typing on a keyboard tray or working with a laptop computer on a lap desk or other surface, your forearms should have the same near parallel relationship to the floor. If your chair has adjustable armrests, fix them so that they support your forearms in a parallel position with the floor. A footrest also helps take the strain off the low back.

The more freedom you have in setting up your workspace, the more back-friendly a routine you can follow. For example, if you have room for a standing desk or a high work counter with a stool, you can vary your working position throughout the day. The variety will be great for your back, decreasing the fatigue and strain that undermine posture and set the stage for injury.

Not everyone can make such choices. Most people have to work at desks and sit in chairs that other people have chosen, maybe with little regard for back health. If that's the case for you, please remember that a varied routine of standing, stretching, and deep breathing at regular intervals throughout the day will do far more to keep your back healthy than even the most ergonomic office.

To make sure you stand up enough, try this trick: Stand when you're on the phone for more than a minute. Standing tall allows you to breathe more deeply, is great for your back, and gives you increased energy that will be heard on the other end of the line as persuasive, compelling confidence.

LIFTING, STOWING, AND OTHER CHORES

Fewer and fewer people in the developed world earn their living doing manual labor. But we still have to mow the lawn, rake the leaves, stow and retrieve seasonal items and clothing, vacuum under the sofa, and carry groceries, toddlers, and laundry around the house, to name just a few common back-sensitive chores.

Developing adequate proprioception and core flexibility, strength, and endurance will help you intuitively keep your body in fluid balance as you perform these tasks. The main principle to follow in lifting, carrying, and other physical work is to keep the top of your head, your ears, shoulders, hips, knees, and ankles aligned in the same plane as much as possible. For example, when stooping down

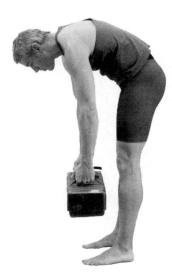

Incorrect lifting posture, with curved back and straight legs, increases the risk of injury.

to pick up a box requires you to break that plane, try to do so as minimally as possible: bend your knees, but keep your back and neck straight and avoid unnecessary twisting motions. Then come fluidly back into alignment as you return to a balanced, upright posture.

If you have to carry bags or other objects in each hand, try to equalize the load. If you have a heavy shoulder bag, regularly shift it from shoulder to shoulder so that you don't overstress one side of your back.

When you have to do a repetitive physical task like shoveling snow or raking leaves, prepare yourself to do it safely by taking a few minutes to stand tall and adjust your breathing. Picture the motions you're going to be making in your mind, and imagine yourself doing them in a graceful, easy rhythm. Every twenty minutes or so, take a break to reset both your breathing and your visualization. These steps will keep you focused and decrease your fatigue as you work, which will make doing the chore faster and safer.

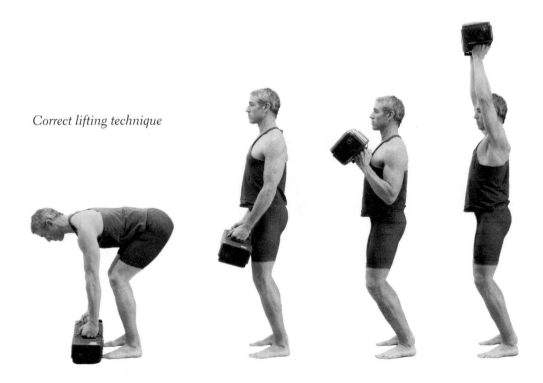

Correct lifting technique

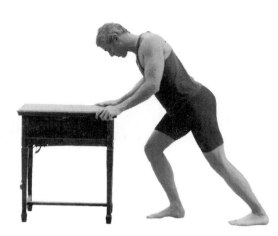

Incorrect pushing

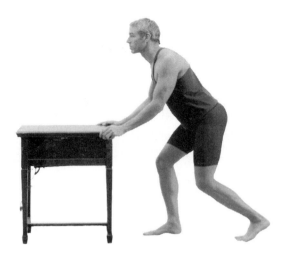

Correct pushing

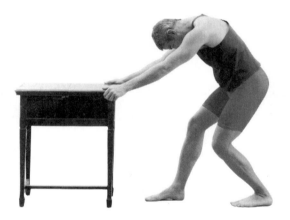

Incorrect pulling

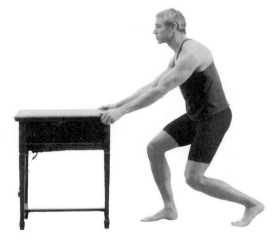

Correct pulling

FITNESS AND SPORTS

A pain-free back is essential to enjoying fitness and sports activities. Back Rx can help by giving you the flexibility, strength, endurance, and balance you need to find healthy, rather than unhealthy, stress in the repetitions of a weight workout or in the acceleration and deceleration of explosive forces in a golf swing or tennis stroke. It can also help you in other ways.

You can use Back Rx's focused breathing and visualization techniques to pace your workout or practice session and give it flow. Set your breath in a full, even rhythm before you begin a practice routine or a new set of repetitions in a workout. While you're setting the breath, visualize yourself rhythmically making the perfect swing or other desired movement. The combination of the focused breath and the guiding image will hone your timing, technique, and form.

Do the same thing when you're on the golf course or tennis court. In between swings or points, refocus your breathing in a full, even rhythm. In addition to helping you make the next shot a better one, this will lessen the risk of injury by keeping you fresh and alert. Recreational sports injuries often begin with a fatigue-induced breakdown in technique.

GOLF

Few activities stress the back as much as golf. Even if you have sound technique, your back must be supple and strong to withstand the repetitive force of the golf swing. Back Rx Series A or B can be a great warm-up for a round of golf. You may also like to add these specific pre-golf stretches, which are demonstrated by Sara Bartlett, a physical therapist for the Ladies Professional Golf Association (LPGA). Hold each stretch for five breaths, three times.

HAMSTRING/CALF STRETCH

- Lean into a wall or other support with straight arms. Keeping your back and neck straight, press forward as if you were trying to walk the wall backward, with one leg bent and the other leg straight behind you. You should feel the stretch in the hamstring and calf of the straight leg. Hold the stretch for at least five deep breaths in and out.
- Repeat with other leg straight.

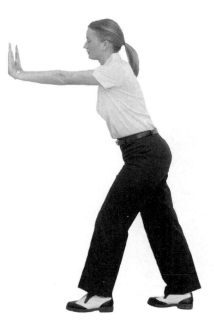

PARASPINAL STRETCH

- Stand as if you are ready to address the ball, bending forward slightly at the hips while keeping your back and neck straight. Loop your forearms around a club behind your back, and slowly twist back and forth for at least five deep breaths in and out.

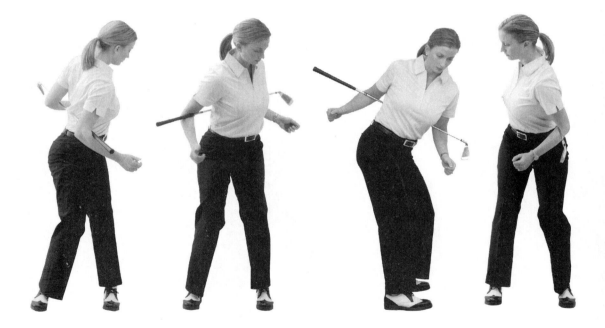

SHOULDER/HIP STRETCH

- Lie flat on your back and bend the left leg so that the foot rests above your right knee.
- Reach across your chest with your left arm, and pull gently on the elbow with your right hand. Hold the stretch for at least five deep breaths in and out.
- Repeat with opposite arm and leg.

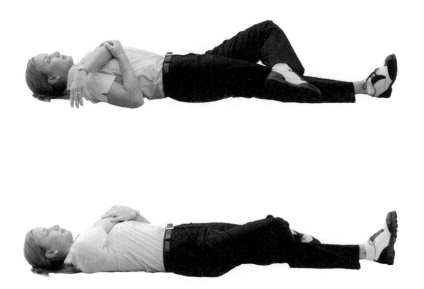

ILIOTIBIAL BAND STRETCH

- Lie flat on your back with your legs straight and your arms extended to the sides.
- Slowly raise one leg into a bent-knee position with the foot flat on the floor on the outside of your other knee.
- Let gravity pull your bent knee toward the floor on the outside of the straight leg. Hold the stretch for at least five deep breaths in and out.
- Repeat with other leg.

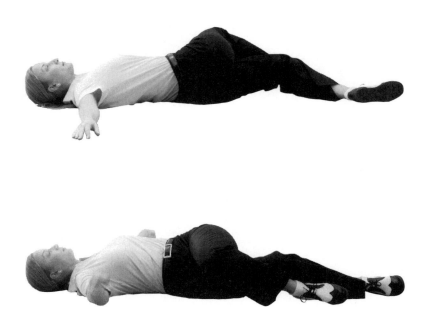

PIRIFORMIS STRETCH

- Lie flat on your back with your knees bent and your feet flat on the floor.
- Raise the right foot to rest against the left knee.
- Clasp your hands behind the bent left knee and pull gently toward your chest. Hold the stretch for at least five deep breaths in and out.
- Repeat with other leg.

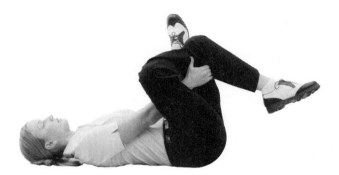

STRESS MANAGEMENT

The focused breathing skills learned in Back Rx can relieve stress in two ways. When a tense situation occurs and fear, anxiety, anger, or other difficult emotions threaten to get the better of you, tuning in to your breathing and giving it a deep, even rhythm can calm you enough to make it through the tough times.

Regular sessions of focused breathing during the day, on the other hand, can keep you on a more even keel in the first place. In this regard, don't let yourself get caught in time traps. Even when you feel you are running nonstop, there are empty moments during the day when you can calm and center yourself. If you have ten minutes between appointments, or before you have to pick up the kids at soccer practice, seize five of them to practice the controlled breathing of Back Rx.

You can do this almost anywhere, anytime. But please don't do it while you're driving your car. If you need to take a stress-reduction break in the car, pull over and park first. Then when you get back on the road, you'll have the advantage of greater alertness and calm to help you drive defensively and safely.

AIRLINE TRAVEL

As if sitting down in a cramped airline seat for a lengthy period weren't bad enough, traveling in a pressurized cabin subjects the discs to added pressure. And over the course of the flight, the recirculating air in the cabin gets staler and staler, and lower in nourishing oxygen. It's almost as if commercial airline travel were designed to trigger low back episodes.

There are a few things you can do to protect your back when you fly. If your back has been problematic recently, take two or three Advil or other anti-inflammatories before the flight. Drink plenty of water to keep yourself as hydrated as possible. And, especially on long flights, stand up periodically to stretch and walk up and down the aisle. Ideally, you should do this every twenty to thirty minutes, following the same schedule you use to keep your back calm at the office.

CHAPTER SIX

RESUMING ACTIVITY AFTER A LOW BACK INJURY

For the first two to three days after a low back injury, restrict your activities and stay home to rest and recuperate. If you keep pushing yourself, you will only make your recovery slower and less complete. During this time, you should take modified bed rest. This means spending most of the day resting quietly in the most comfortable position you can find. The two positions that work best for most people are on the side in a slightly fetal position with a pillow between the knees, or flat on the back with the legs raised. The second position helps the lower back muscles to relax because it takes the strain of gravity off them. These are also generally the best positions for sleeping at night.

Don't spend all day in bed, however. Uninterrupted bed rest can be counterproductive. If you are confined to bed completely, you will lose 1% of your muscle mass each day. Instead, get up every hour or couple of hours to walk around a little and arch backward. You can also try some light stretching, by pulling each knee up to your chest for a moment or two. Go just to the point where the strain is about to become intense, stop there, and take two or three slow, controlled breaths. This is also a good idea if you find you can't sleep through the whole night, which is often the case when a low back injury is fresh.

During the first couple of days, avoid chair-sitting as much as possible. When you do sit down, make sure that you stand up after fifteen or twenty minutes to straighten your back and arch it backward a little.

You should also avoid lifting anything heavy. This can be an especially difficult rule to follow if you have young children who want to be lifted and held, but do your best. It may seem a little hard-hearted in the short term, but it will help you achieve your goal of becoming pain-free so you can lift your child to your heart's content. If you undermine your recovery with inappropriate activity and stress, your back pain will keep you from being the parent you want to be for longer than is absolutely necessary.

After two to three days of this modified bed rest, you should be ready to walk and stretch gently for longer periods. By doing so, you prepare the body for greater activity and prime the release of endorphins, the body's natural opiates, which will lessen your reliance on pain medication and improve your healing.

These guidelines apply to everyone with low back pain except seniors. During acute back pain episodes, seniors should minimize their walking. Stationary bicycling is much better for seniors because it is a gentle, nonimpact activity and carries a lower risk of falls.

In addition, everyone with low back pain, of every age and physical condition, can benefit enormously from aquatherapy. Your buoyancy in the water will take all the stress off your back. Wear a flotation vest or belt and gently do a cycling motion with your legs. This relaxed, stress-free, floating movement will do wonders for your back and your peace of mind. Well-conditioned athletes usually hop in the pool for aquatherapy no later than the day after they hurt themselves.

After a week or so of alternating rest with gradually increasing activity, you should be ready to start the Back Rx exercises. But don't worry if it takes a little longer. The most important thing is to move at your own pace. If you feel ready to do more before the week is out, that's fine. But in general, a slow and steady start leads to better healing.

To illustrate how Back Rx can help you beat low back pain and reactivate your lifestyle, I'd like to tell you about two typical patients. One used the program to recover from an acute injury. The other used it to break a long cycle of chronic pain.

Stacy M., a law student in her early twenties, came to see me when she experienced intense back pain and was diagnosed with an acute disc herniation a week after taking her first-year final exams. She was worried that the injury might ruin her whole summer, including an important internship at a law firm.

Stacy was in good health. She was not overweight. And she had no complicating conditions.

Fortunately, she had a little flexibility in beginning her internship, and she arranged to postpone the start of it for one month. For the first couple of days, she did nothing but rest and use ibuprofen, heat, and ice to ease her pain and inflammation. When she wasn't lying down in the least painful position possible, she minimized her sitting, getting up every fifteen or twenty minutes to stand straight and tall and arch backward. As she felt able to, she walked around a little, or lay down on her back on the floor to pull each knee up to her chest in turn. Every half hour or so, she also made an effort to focus her attention on her breathing, slowing it down and making it fuller and deeper, often doing so in combination with a light stretch.

Within seven days, she felt well enough to begin the Back Rx exercises.

After a month of Back Rx, she was pain-free and ready to start her internship and enjoy the rest of her summer.

Most acute pain episodes will respond to the Back Rx program just as well. But everyone will progress on an individual schedule. The important thing is not how fast you move through each stage of recovery, but that you continue to experience steady, gradual improvement. Sooner or later you will turn the corner, if you stick with the program.

Chronic pain patients dispense with the bed rest stage and immediately begin doing the Back Rx exercises, moving slowly and surely at an individual pace. If you suffer chronic pain from a series of back injuries or years of overuse and neglect, it may take quite a while to achieve 100% recovery. But the progress you make in the short term can vastly improve your quality of life.

Father X, a Connecticut clergyman in his mid-forties, consulted me after almost twenty years of debilitating low back pain. His problems were exacerbated by his high weight and low fitness level, two common conditions for someone unable to move without pain for years. To function at all he was taking six Percocets and four Valium every single day. Despite the daily pain, and the assurances of many doctors that surgery was the only option left, he was determined to avoid invasive procedures.

I encouraged Father X to make a fresh start with the Back Rx program and to adjust his diet. He also took advantage of his access to a pool to do aquatherapy. Although he had mildly increased symptoms for the first few weeks, as is common in some cases, I encouraged him to stick with the program.

Six months later, Father X had lost weight and significantly raised his fitness level and his spirits. He still had some back pain, but much less than before. For the first time in twenty years, pain no longer dominated every waking moment. He was able to cut his daily dose of Percocet in half, and to stop taking Valium. That in itself greatly improved his quality of life. Moreover, his progress kept him motivated to stay with the program and he continued to improve steadily.

These are the sorts of results that Back Rx regularly helps patients to achieve. If you've had an acute injury and have rested up a little, or if you've been suffering from chronic pain, it's time to begin the exercises and get yourself started on the same road to recovery.

PART TWO

BACK Rx SERIES A, B, AND C

CHAPTER SEVEN

INTRODUCTION:
DOING THE BACK Rx EXERCISES

Back Rx Series A, B, and C all develop flexibility, strength, and endurance with elements of physical therapy and rehabilitation, yoga, and Pilates. But each series has its own special emphasis and its own distinctive recipe. The breakdown looks like this:

	PHYSICAL THERAPY/REHABILITATION	YOGA	PILATES
Series A	50%	30%	20%
Series B	30%	50%	20%
Series C	20%	30%	50%

Series A emphasizes isometric muscle work derived from physical therapy to lay a foundation of core muscle flexibility and prepare the body for the increased stress of strength and endurance training. Series B takes the healing farther with more yoga-based work that intensifies the isometric loading of core muscles and adds more dynamic muscle work to build strength through concentric, eccentric, and plyometric contractions. Series C maximizes endurance training with an expanded Pilates component that makes the routine an almost continuous plyometric work-out for the body's core muscles.

As I've mentioned, although full-scale yoga and Pilates are ultimately the best methods for maximizing back health, they both contain positions and movements that can easily traumatize a weak back. The yoga- and Pilates-based elements of Back Rx have been modified to eliminate these extreme stresses. What remains is a hallmark of both yoga and Pilates, the combination of targeted muscle work with proper breath control.

The ancient yogists closely observed how the mind and breath influence each other. When we are agitated, our breathing accelerates and becomes more shallow. When we are calm, our breathing slows and deepens. From this starting point, the various yoga postures for meditation and physical development evolved to facilitate breathing and carry its benefits throughout the body.

The scientific basis of yoga's effectiveness is that the yoga postures and controlled breathing deliver elevated levels of oxygen to nourish muscles, ligaments, tendons, and other tissues in a precise way. Hatha-Yoga (pronounced "hut-ta"), the physical training that is yoga's most familiar face in the Western world, may perhaps best be understood as the practice of forceful breathing.

Likewise with Pilates. Although Pilates exercises stand on their own as an integrated movement and body practice, Joseph Pilates (1880–1967) made no secret of the inspiration and insight he found in yoga. He regularly took yoga postures and their carefully controlled breathing as a starting point, and then added dynamic plyometric muscle work to accelerate each posture's ability to enhance flexibility, strength, and endurance.

If you're interested in doing nonmedical yoga and Pilates, the medical yoga and medical Pilates of Back Rx will get you in shape to benefit from them. You'll be ready to move on to full-scale yoga or Pilates when you can do Back Rx Series B totally pain-free.

As with any exercise program, it is a good idea to get your doctor's okay before beginning Back Rx. After that, feel free to move through the sequence of the A, B, and C series at your own pace. But don't jump ahead. You should not attempt Series B until you can do Series A totally pain-free, and you should not attempt Series C — or full-scale yoga or Pilates—until you can do Series B totally pain-free.

Please keep in mind, however, that you can complete the Back Rx program, and achieve a full and lasting recovery, simply by doing Series A. The first series is designed to get you moving again without pain, and many people maintain good back health by continuing to do Series A consistently. But if you do progress to Series B or C, you will reach substantially higher back fitness levels.

Remember, too, that when it comes to the low back, Pain ≠ Gain. If you experience sharp pain at any time, first take a break and then try to do the movement more precisely and gently. You should expect and tolerate a little discomfort, as you press to the limit of your stretch, but not more than that. If sharp pain persists no matter how gingerly you try to do the movement, you should stop doing Back Rx and consult a qualified physician.

That said, here is a typical schedule as a guideline. As you become comfortable doing Back Rx, adjust the schedule to suit your own needs and pace of recovery.

Week One

- If you are recovering from an acute injury, first take two to three days of modified bed rest as explained in Chapter 6.
- Begin Series A by doing the routine every other day, with a rest day in between. If your back feels very tender, do only exercises 1–9 (stopping before "Hip Hikers"). The first eight exercises are all done flat on your back, which minimizes the pressure on deconditioned and injured muscles and discs.

- Move carefully from one position and exercise to another. Quick, jerky movements can easily worsen an existing injury or cause a fresh one.
- The time of day is up to you. If you're a morning person, do the routine in the morning; it will get the day off to a good start. If you're not a morning person, choose another time; an evening session of Back Rx, for example, is a great way to shed the pressures of the day so that you can get a decent night's rest.
- To maximize the benefit of any Back Rx routine, apply moist heat in the shower or with a heating pad for up to thirty minutes before you do the exercises, and apply ice for fifteen minutes afterward.

Weeks Two to Three

- Continue doing Series A every other day, with a rest day in between. If you have begun by doing only the first eight exercises, gradually build to doing the full Series A routine.

Weeks Three to Four

- Begin to increase the frequency of your workouts by doing Series A two days in a row, and then taking a rest day.
- Gradually build to doing the full Series A for fifteen minutes every day.

Week Five

- Begin Series B by doing the routine every other day with a rest day in between.
- Or continue doing Series A.

Weeks Six to Eight

- Gradually build to doing Series B every day.
- Or continue doing Series A.

- To sustain your recovery and minimize recurrences, continue doing Series A or Series B regularly, at least three times a week.
- Or begin Series C by doing the routine every other day with a rest day in between. Gradually build to doing Series C for fifteen minutes every day. When you have reached the point where you can do Series C comfortably every day, you can decrease the frequency to three times a week, if you like, and still maintain your new fitness level.

Many people like to work out while listening to music. But I suggest doing the Back Rx workouts without any music on at first, so that you can concentrate on your breathing and learn to control it properly. Tuning your senses in to your own body's signals, including the distinctive sound of your own healthy breathing, requires regular doses of silence.

But as you get comfortable doing the Back Rx routines, add some music to support a good workout rhythm, if you like. All sorts of music can work well with Back Rx, so long as it's music that you enjoy. Just do your body and mind a favor and try some nice gentle sambas before you start rocking yourself around too frenetically. If you've found working with guided imagery helpful, music can become a soundtrack for those images and magnify their healing impact.

As you follow the Back Rx program, it's a good idea to keep track of your progress on a weekly basis. (A day is too short a time frame to measure: some days will go better than others; and minor setbacks will almost always occur here and there.) Take a few minutes to assess how you've felt and functioned, using a scale from 1 to 10, where 1 is miserable and 10 is great. Try to make each week's assessment without referring to the previous weeks' scores so that they don't bias you.

In the first few weeks of the program, you may experience mildly increased symptoms. This is normal, and you shouldn't let it keep you from doing the exercises.

To minimize any temporary mild increase in your symptoms, apply heat before doing the exercises and ice afterward.

If you follow the Back Rx program faithfully, you will almost certainly see your scores go up week by week. Seeing your progress quantified can provide powerful motivation to stick with the program and achieve full recovery. It also serves as an early warning system to help you take corrective action and head off more serious problems. That could mean re-committing yourself to the Back Rx program and/or seeking professional help to bolster your efforts.

In the vast majority of cases, however, Back Rx will be all you need to rediscover the joy of a healthy back and pain-free movement. I recommend starting Back Rx after clearing it with a physician; if your pain increases suddenly or does not improve after eight weeks of Back Rx, you should seek a physician's advice. Now let's look closely at how to do the exercises in each series.

CHAPTER EIGHT

RETURN TO MOVEMENT:
BACK Rx SERIES A

Back Rx Series A will help you get moving again without pain. Hold each posture for five full breaths.

SUN SALUTATION LYING DOWN

The Sun Salutation Lying Down is a variation of the standing Sun Salutation with which yoga practitioners have greeted the day for thousands of years. The most important modification is that the exercise is done flat on your back. The first half of the Series A routine is done in the same position to maximize support for, and minimize pressure on, the low back and the lumbar vertebral discs.

To do the Sun Salutation Lying Down:

- Lie flat on your back with your legs straight and your arms straight and long at your sides. Look up at the ceiling, so that your neck and back form one continuous line.

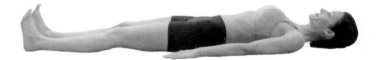

- Inhale as you sweep your arms out from your sides along the floor to point above your head. Imagine the line of your neck and spine becoming even longer and straighter.

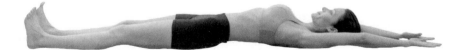

- Keeping your arms straight, sweep them up behind your head toward the ceiling and slowly let gravity pull them back to your sides, with your palms flat on the floor. Exhale slowly and fully as you do this.

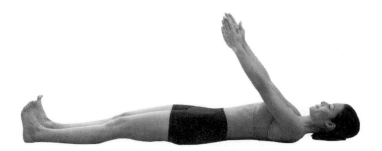

The Sun Salutation Lying Down is a warm-up stretch that prepares the body for action and sets the breathing tempo for all of Series A. If you like, you can do a series of Sun Salutations Lying Down until you feel your breathing settle into a slow, even tempo. Then you're ready to begin Series A in earnest.

BRIDGING

- Slowly raise your knees, one leg at a time, to a bent position with your feet flat on the floor. Point the feet straight ahead or put them in a slightly pigeon-toed position. Bridging works the lower abdominal and low back area, and it opens up and stretches the hip flexors. A slightly pigeon-toed stance will put more focus on the abdominal region; straight toes will put a little more pressure on your gluteal and inner-thigh muscles. Don't point your toes out, as this can put excessive strain on your knees.

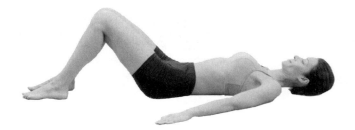

- Take a slow deep breath in, then tighten your buttocks and pull in your abdominal muscles, so that your hips roll upward. Exhale slowly and fully as your hips come off the floor. It is not important to lift the hips very high to start; just getting them off the floor is enough as you become accustomed to the movement. As you grow more comfortable with the routine, you can gradually increase the height.

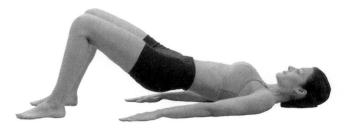

- Hold the position for five deep breaths. That means five full inhalations and five full exhalations. This should take about fifteen seconds, depending on your lung capacity. But don't watch the clock. Concentrate on breathing in the same slow, even tempo that you established in the Sun Salutation. Hold the posture, but never hold your breath. Continuous, flowing breathing drives oxygen to the body areas that the exercise is targeting.
- Relax as you begin to take your sixth breath, and gently let your hips down to the floor. Don't drop your hips abruptly like a sack of potatoes. You want a controlled descent, as if your body were sinking slowly through a pool of water or Jell-O.
- Perform another Sun Salutation Lying Down to relax your body completely and re-establish a good breathing tempo.

ABDOMINAL CRUNCH

- Lie on the floor on your back with your arms at your sides and your palms flat on the floor, and then slowly raise one knee at a time to a bent position, with your feet flat on the floor.
- Inhale fully as you raise your shoulders off the floor and squeeze your abdominals. Don't raise your head first. Instead, try to keep your neck straight and let your head come up off the floor with your shoulders. If you lift your head high enough to bend your neck forward, you will not only work the abdominals less, but you will also slightly constrict your breathing and risk straining your neck muscles.

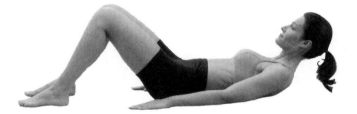

- Exhale slowly, then take four more full breaths, in and out, while you hold the stretch.
- Throughout the stretch, keep your palms, the insides of your forearms, and your elbows in contact with the floor. This focuses the exertion on isometrically contracting the oblique and upper abdominal muscles and on loosening up the hip flexors.

- Relax back to the starting position as you take a sixth full breath.
- Straighten one leg at a time from the bent-knee position, and perform another Sun Salutation Lying Down.

KNEE TO CHEST

This exercise increases the stress on your abdominal muscles and begins to stretch them dynamically as well as isometrically.

- Lie on your back with your arms straight and long at your sides, your knees bent, and your feet flat on the floor. Point your toes straight ahead or turn them in slightly toward each other.
- Clasp your hands in the crook of one bent knee, and gently pull the knee toward your chest. Inhale slowly and fully as you reach the limit of your stretch, and raise your shoulders just off the floor to help open up the hip flexor. Point the toes of the raised foot toward the ceiling and try to hold your raised leg parallel to the floor, as if you were balancing a teacup on the top of your shin.

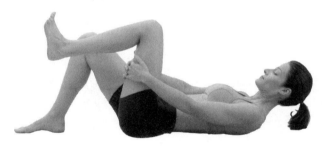

- Exhale slowly, then hold the position at full stretch for four more deep breaths in and out.
- Relax back to the starting position as you take the sixth breath.

- Repeat the stretch with the other knee pulled to your chest.
- Perform a Sun Salutation Lying Down.

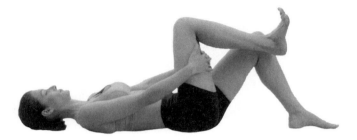

ABDOMINAL CRUNCH WITH LEG FLEXED

- Lie flat on your back with your arms at your sides, palms on the floor. Gently raise one knee into a bent position while keeping the other leg straight, with the toes of the straight leg pointing to the ceiling.
- Inhale fully and gently raise your chest by bringing your shoulders off the floor. Keep your neck straight to facilitate breathing and try to raise your head and shoulders as one unit, or let your head lag slightly after your shoulders.

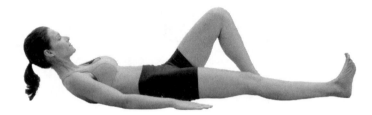

- Exhale slowly and hold the posture for four more full breaths in and out.
- Relax back to the starting position, gently lowering your shoulders to the floor as you take a sixth breath.

• Repeat the stretch with the other knee bent, then perform another Sun Salutation Lying Down.

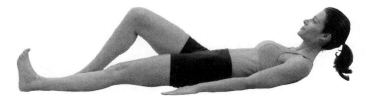

TREE POSE

With the Tree Pose you're beginning to work the full hip musculature, including the hip flexors, abductors, external rotators, and extensors. In physical therapy, this is known as a classic FABERE (Flexion, Abduction, External Rotation, and Extension) stretch. The continuous breathing that Back Rx adds to the stretch maximizes its benefit by driving more oxygen to the hip and pelvic area.

- Lie flat on your back with your arms at your sides, palms facing down.
- As you inhale slowly and deeply, bend one leg and place the sole of that foot on the inside of your other knee. If you can't comfortably bring the sole of the foot as high as the knee, rest it against the inside of the lower leg.

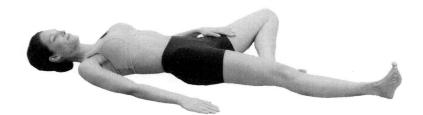

- Exhale slowly, and hold the position for four more full breaths in and out.
- Look straight up at the ceiling and imagine your spine and neck lengthening in one continuous line.
- Relax back to the starting position as you take a sixth breath.

- Repeat the stretch with the other leg bent and then perform another Sun Salutation Lying Down.

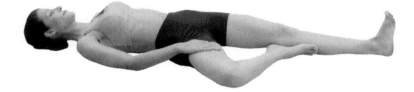

BOUND ANGLE POSTURE

The Bound Angle Posture is a FABERE stretch for both hips at once.

- Lie flat on your back with your arms at your sides, palms down.
- As you inhale slowly, draw one foot at a time in toward your groin, so that your heels touch but your toes do not.

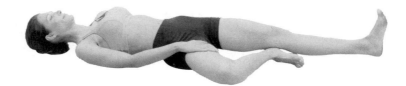

- Exhale slowly, and focus on the feeling of gravity pulling your knees to the floor. Imagine your knees spreading apart from each other like the opening of an Oriental fan. Keeping your heels together and making a "V" with your feet works in symbiosis with the knees to open up the hips.

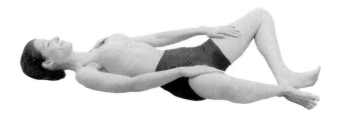

- Hold the position for four more full breaths in and out.
- Relax to the starting position, slowly straightening your legs one at a time, as you take a sixth breath. Then do another Sun Salutation Lying Down.

LUMBAR ROTATION DOUBLE KNEE

This posture works the abdominal obliques and begins to stretch the Ilio-Tibial-Band (ITB), which runs along the outside of your hip and thigh. The ITB is crucial to flexibility, and a tight ITB can cause sciatic symptoms. The Lumbar Rotation Double Knee also begins to stretch the paraspinal muscles, which run up and down both sides of the spine. As Back Rx Series A continues, it gradually works more and more of the areas that are important for the back's flexibility, strength, and endurance.

- Lie on your back with your knees bent and feet flat on the floor, and extend your arms straight out from your shoulders.

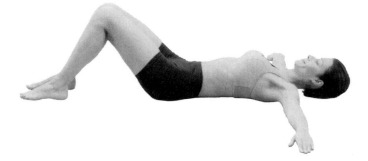

- Inhale fully, and slowly lower your knees to one side, while keeping your shoulders flat to the floor. Don't force your knees down to the side. Let gravity do the work.

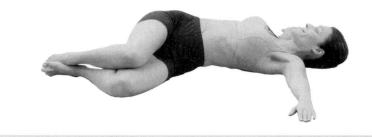

- Exhale, then hold the position for four more breaths in and out.
- Raise your knees back to the starting position as you take a sixth breath.
- Repeat the stretch by lowering your knees to the other side.
- Perform another Sun Salutation Lying Down.

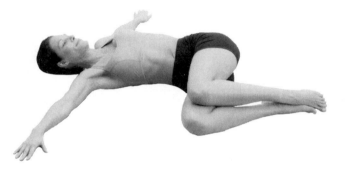

LUMBAR ROTATION SINGLE KNEE

This exercise increases the stretch of the ITB and the paraspinal muscles.

- After you finish the last Sun Salutation Lying Down, slowly turn onto one side and support your head on one hand. Place the other hand palm down in front of your chest and lean into it gently for support.

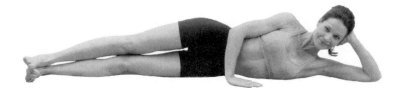

- Inhale fully, and cross your top leg over the bottom one so that your bent knee touches the floor in front of you at about waist height and your foot rests on the floor in front of the knee of your straight lower leg.

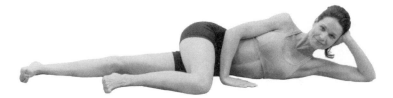

- Exhale, and hold the position for four more breaths in and out.
- Release the posture and turn gently onto your back as you take a sixth breath.
- Repeat on the other side, then do another Sun Salutation Lying Down.

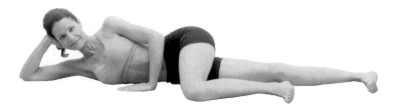

HIP HIKERS

The Hip Hikers exercise helps to maximize the range of motion in your hips and is the most strenuous FABERE stretch in Series A. It concludes the supine warm-up period of the workout. The remaining exercises will be a little more heavy-duty.

- Take the same starting position as in the Lumbar Rotation Single Knee, lying on one side with one hand holding up your head and the other placed in front of your chest to support your whole body at a slight angle toward the floor.
- Keeping both legs straight, slowly raise one leg as you inhale fully.

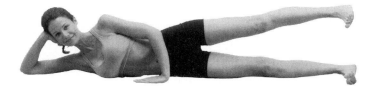

- Exhale, and hold the position for four more full breaths in and out, feeling the stretch in your hip and thigh.
- Gently lower the leg as you take a sixth breath.
- Repeat on the other side, then do another Sun Salutation Lying Down.

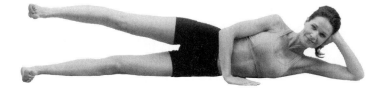

STAFF POSTURE

The Staff Posture gives you an increased paraspinal stretch, opens up the chest, pectoral muscles, and shoulders, and flexes the hamstrings and quadriceps.

- After the last Sun Salutation Lying Down, slowly and gently move into a seated position on the floor with your legs straight out in front of you, toes pointed to the ceiling, and your hands positioned slightly behind your hips for support, palms flat on the floor. If you find it difficult to keep your legs straight, it is okay to let them bend a bit.

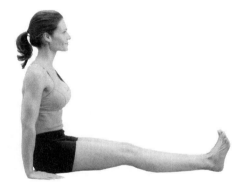

- Keeping your back and neck as straight as possible, so that they form one continuous line, take five full breaths in and out. Arch your back a little, if that feels more comfortable, as this will further decrease pressure on the discs.
- Relax as you take a sixth breath.

SUN SALUTATION ON KNEES

- Carefully move into a kneeling position, with shoulders, hips, and thighs all in line with each other and your hands hanging relaxed at your sides.
- Inhale fully as you sweep your straight arms up at the sides to reach for the ceiling above your head. Keep your back and neck in one lengthening line, so that your gaze is straight in front of you, as if you are looking toward a distant horizon.
- Sweep your straight arms down in front of you to your sides, exhaling slowly as you do so.

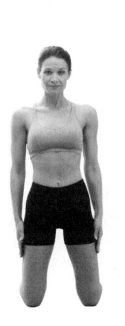
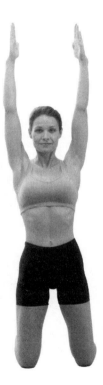

LOCUST POSTURE

This posture works both the paraspinal muscles and the abdominal muscles.

- Carefully move into a prone position, lying flat on the floor on your stomach with your arms straight and long at your sides.
- Keeping your knees straight, raise one leg off the floor as you inhale fully. You should feel the stretch in your hip. It does not matter how high you raise the leg, as long as you keep it straight and the knee is off the floor.

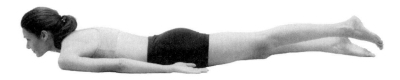

- Try to remain as relaxed as possible in the upper body, and hold the position while taking four more full breaths in and out.
- Relax back to the starting position as you take a sixth breath.
- Repeat the exercise with the other leg, then do a Sun Salutation on Knees.

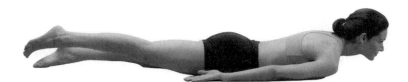

BACK EXTENSION

- Take a position on all fours, with your weight distributed evenly on your hands and knees.

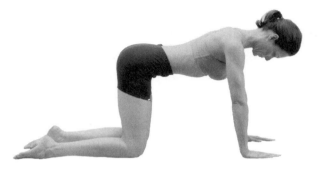

- Keeping your neck and back in line with each other, lift one leg and extend it backward as you inhale fully. Try to feel your neck and back lengthening into one continuous line with the extended leg. Don't cant or tip the hip of the extended leg out of parallel with the other hip, as that will put excessive strain on the canted side. Keeping the hips at the same level applies gentle, healing stress evenly across the whole back.

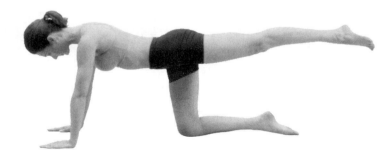

- Exhale slowly, then hold the position for four more breaths in and out.
- Relax back to the starting position on hands and knees as you take a sixth breath.
- Check to make sure your weight is once again distributed evenly on all fours, then repeat the posture by extending the other leg.
- Perform a Sun Salutation on Knees.

CAT STRETCH

The Cat Stretch combines a low back stretch with abdominal contractions and a pelvic tilt.

- Take the same starting position as in Back Extension, with your weight balanced evenly on your hands and knees.
- As you inhale, arch your back as if you are trying to touch the ceiling with the center of your back.

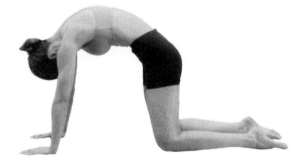

- Exhale, and hold the arched position for four more breaths in and out.

- Then let gravity pull your belly button toward the floor as you continue to breathe slowly and evenly. Hold this position for five full breaths in and out.

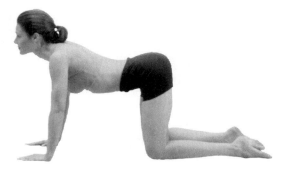

- Relax back to the starting position as you take an eleventh breath.
- Perform a Sun Salutation on Knees.

FLEXIBILITY PRAYER

The Flexibility Prayer introduces weight-bearing stretches of the paraspinal muscles, along with hip rotation and engagement of the oblique abdominal muscles.

- Stand up carefully with your feet the same width apart as your shoulder blades. Let your arms hang easily at your sides and try to make one continuous line of your spine and the back of your neck.
- Stretch your arms out in front of you with your palms together as if in prayer.
- Slowly turn your body as far as you can to one side as you inhale fully.
- Exhale, and hold the position for four more breaths in and out.
- Slowly face front. Then turn to the other side, and hold the position for five more deep breaths in and out.
- Relax back to the starting position with your arms at your sides.

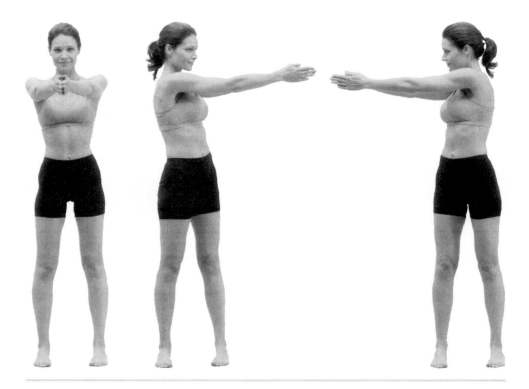

SUN SALUTATION STANDING

- Take the same starting position as in the Flexibility Prayer, standing straight and tall with your feet about the same width apart as your shoulder blades.
- Sweep your arms up to the sides and above your head as you inhale fully.
- Sweep your straight arms down in front of you to return to rest at your sides as you exhale slowly.

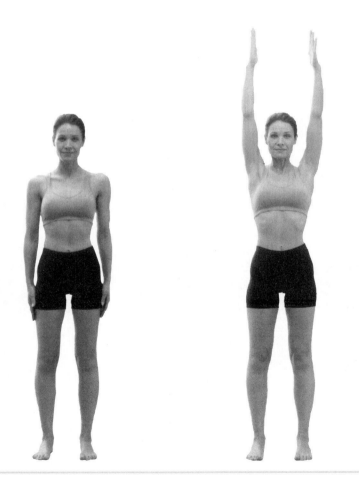

STANDING TREE POSE

This difficult posture fires all the core muscle groups in proper sequence. Don't try to hold the posture for five full breaths when you first do it. Start with three breaths and work your way up.

- Stand straight and tall with your feet about the same width apart as your shoulder blades. Keep your neck straight so that you are looking directly in front of you, as if at a distant horizon.

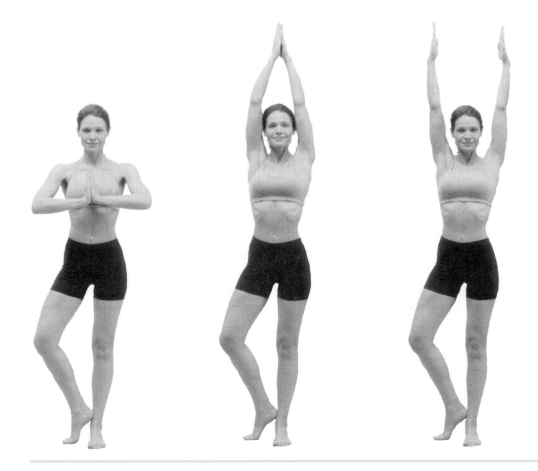

- Bring the heel of one foot up to rest on the ankle of the other leg, with the ball of the foot continuing to touch the floor.
- Inhale slowly as you raise your arms to reach for the sky.
- Exhale slowly, and take two more deep breaths in and out.
- Relax to the starting position as you take a fourth full breath.
- Repeat with the other heel raised to rest on your other ankle.
- Perform a Sun Salutation Standing.

Congratulations! You've now completed Back Rx Series A.

CHAPTER NINE

RESUMING FULL ACTIVITY: BACK Rx SERIES B

Back Rx Series B will help you complete your recovery and return to an active lifestyle. The Series B exercises build on the Series A exercises in two ways. The postures themselves are a little more difficult, and the routine calls for holding every posture for seven full breaths instead of five.

SUN SALUTATION LYING DOWN

- Lie flat on your back with your legs straight and your arms straight and long at your sides. Look straight up at the ceiling so that your neck and back form one continuous line.

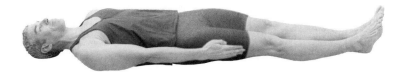

- Sweep your arms out from your sides along the floor to point straight back above your head. Inhale as you do, so that the lungs fill completely as your arms point straight back behind you. Imagine the straight line of your neck and spine becoming even longer and straighter.

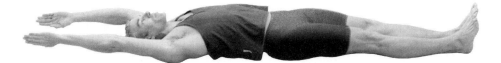

- Keeping your arms straight, sweep them up behind your head to the ceiling and slowly let gravity carry them back to your sides, with your palms flat to the floor. Exhale slowly and fully as you do this.

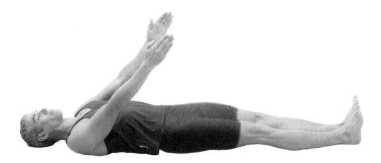

INTERMEDIATE BRIDGING

- Lie flat on your back on the floor, with your arms at your sides, palms down. Slowly raise your knees, one leg at a time, to a bent position with your feet flat on the floor. Point your feet straight ahead or put them in a slightly pigeon-toed position. A pigeon-toed stance will put more focus on the abdominal region; straight toes put more pressure on your gluteal and inner-thigh muscles.

- Take a slow deep breath in, tightening your buttocks and pulling in your abdominal muscles, so that your hips roll upward. Exhale slowly and fully as your hips come off the floor.

- Series A only required lifting the hips off the floor. Series B is more strenuous, and here the aim is to raise the hips and pelvis in line with the thighs.

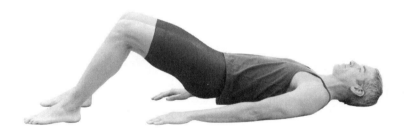

- Hold the position for seven deep breaths in and out. This should take twenty seconds or so, depending on your lung capacity. But don't watch the clock. Concentrate on breathing in the same slow even tempo that you established in the Sun Salutation. Hold the posture, but never hold your breath. Continuous, flowing breathing drives oxygen to the areas of the body that the exercise is targeting.

- Relax as you take an eighth breath, and gently let your hips down to the floor. Don't let your hips drop all at once like a sack of potatoes. You want a controlled descent, as if your body were sinking slowly through a pool of water or Jell-O.

Perform another Sun Salutation Lying Down to relax your body completely and reestablish a good breathing tempo.

INTERMEDIATE ABDOMINAL CRUNCH

In this posture and the ones immediately following, crossing your arms on your chest, instead of resting them on the floor at your sides, will isolate the abdominal muscles and work them harder than the corresponding Series A postures.

- Lie on the floor on your back with your arms crossed on your chest, and then slowly raise one knee at a time to a bent position, with your feet flat on the floor.
- Inhale fully as you raise your shoulders off the floor and squeeze your abdominals. Don't raise your head first. Instead, try to keep your neck straight and let your head and shoulders come up off the floor as a unit.
- Exhale slowly, then take six more full breaths, in and out, while you hold the stretch.
- Relax back to the starting position as you take an eighth full breath.
- Straighten one leg at a time from the bent knee position, and perform another Sun Salutation Lying Down.

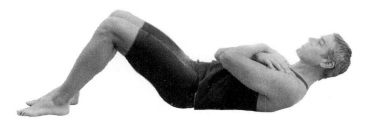

KNEE TO CHEST WITH LEG STRAIGHT

- Lie flat on your back with your arms crossed over your chest and your legs straight. Flex your legs so that your toes point straight to the ceiling.
- Lift one knee and bring it as close to your chest as possible. Inhale slowly and fully as you press to the limit of your stretch, and raise your shoulders just off the floor to help open up the hip flexor. Point the toes of the raised foot toward the ceiling and try to hold your raised leg parallel to the floor, as if you were balancing a teacup on the top of your shin.

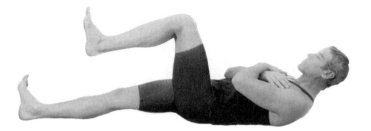

- Exhale slowly, then hold the position at full stretch for six more deep breaths in and out.
- Relax back to the starting position as you take your eighth breath.
- Repeat the stretch with the other knee pulled to your chest.
- Perform a Sun Salutation Lying Down.

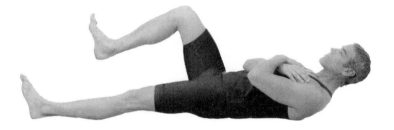

INTERMEDIATE ABDOMINAL CRUNCH WITH LEG FLEXED

- Lie flat on your back with your arms crossed on your chest. Gently raise one knee into a bent position. Lift the other leg, keeping it flexed straight, until your thighs are parallel with each other.

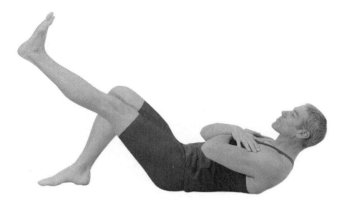

- Inhale fully, and gently raise your chest by bringing your shoulders off the floor. Keep your neck straight to facilitate breathing, and try to raise your head and shoulders as one unit, or let your head lag slightly after your shoulders.
- Exhale slowly, and hold the posture for six more full breaths in and out.
- Relax back to the starting position, gently lowering your shoulders to the floor as you take an eighth breath.

- Repeat the stretch with the other knee bent, then perform another Sun Salutation Lying Down.

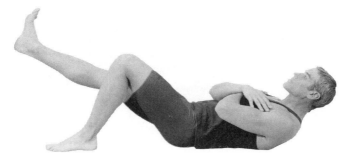

TREE POSE WITH LEG CROSSED

- Lie flat on your back with your arms at your sides, palms facing down.
- As you inhale slowly and deeply, bend one leg and rest that foot on the top of your other knee. This opens up the hip flexor and lets gravity give you more of a stretch than in the Series A Tree Pose.

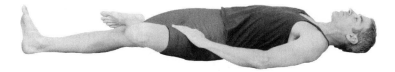

- Exhale slowly, and hold the position for six more full breaths in and out.
- Look straight up at the ceiling and imagine your spine and neck lengthening in one continuous line.
- Relax back to the starting position as you take an eighth breath.
- Repeat the stretch with the other leg bent and then perform another Sun Salutation Lying Down.

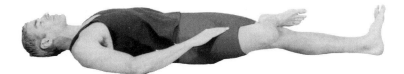

BOUND ANGLE POSTURE WITH FEET TOGETHER

- Lie flat on your back with your arms at your sides, palms down.
- As you inhale slowly, draw one foot at a time in toward your groin, so that the soles of your feet touch. Imagine that the soles of your feet are glued together; this opens up the hip flexors more than the Series A Bound Angle Posture, where the feet form a "V" shape.
- Exhale slowly, and focus on the feeling of gravity pulling your knees to the floor. Imagine your knees spreading apart from each other like the opening of an Oriental fan.
- Hold the position for six more full breaths in and out.
- Relax to the starting position, slowly straightening your legs one at a time, as you take an eighth breath. Then do another Sun Salutation Lying Down.

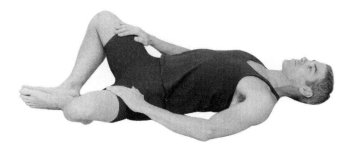

LUMBAR ROTATION WITH LEG CROSSED

- Lie flat on your back with your legs straight and your arms extended straight out to the sides.
- Slowly raise one leg into a bent-knee position with the foot flat on the floor on the outside of your other knee.
- Inhale fully, and let gravity pull your bent knee down to the floor to the outside of the straight leg.

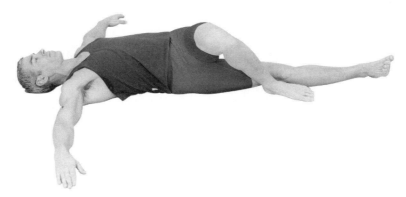

- Exhale slowly, then hold the position for six more deep breaths in and out.
- Relax back to the starting position as you take an eighth breath.
- Repeat with the other knee raised, and then perform another Sun Salutation Lying Down.

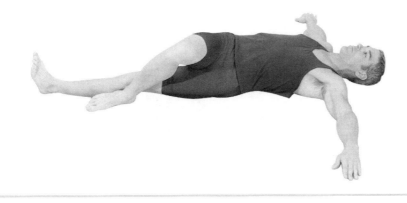

SIDE TREE

- Lie on your side with your head supported by one hand and the other palm flat on the floor in front of your chest, supporting your body.
- Inhale fully as you raise your upper leg into a bent-knee position and rest the sole of that foot on the floor in front of your straight knee.

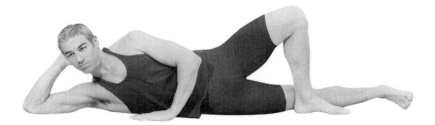

- Exhale slowly, and hold the position for six more deep breaths in and out.
- Relax back to the starting position as you take an eighth breath.
- Carefully turn over onto your other side and repeat the posture with the opposite leg.
- Perform another Sun Salutation Lying Down.

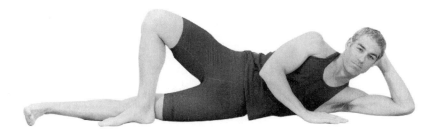

THIGH PULL

- Lie on your side with your head supported by one hand.
- Inhale fully as you reach behind you with the other hand to grasp the ankle of your top leg, and pull your heel toward your buttocks.
- Try to touch your buttocks with your heel. If you can't stretch quite that far at first, that's okay. Work up to it gradually. Concentrate on keeping a smooth straight line down the front of your body, and on keeping your thighs parallel with each other.

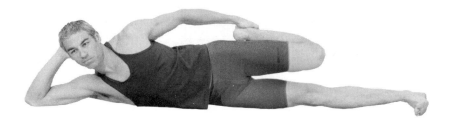

- Exhale slowly, and hold the position for six more deep breaths in and out.
- Relax to the starting position as you take an eighth breath.
- Carefully turn over onto your other side, and repeat the stretch with the opposite leg.
- Do another Sun Salutation Lying Down.

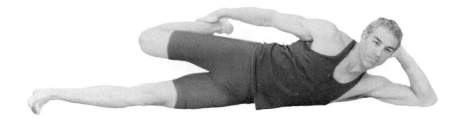

INTERMEDIATE STAFF POSTURE

- After the last Sun Salutation Lying Down, slowly and gently move into a seated position on the floor with your legs straight out in front of you, toes pointed to the ceiling, and your hands positioned beside your hips for support, palms flat on the floor. If you find it difficult to keep your legs straight, it is okay to let them bend a bit. Doing this exercise with your hands beside your hips, rather than behind them as in Series A, imposes a more upright posture that more fully engages the abdominals and the lower back.

- Keeping your back and neck as straight as possible, so that they form one continuous line, take seven full breaths in and out. Arch your back a little, if that feels more comfortable, as this will further decrease pressure on the discs.

- Relax as you take an eighth breath.

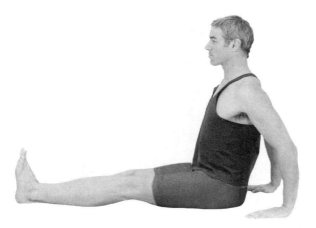

SUN SALUTATION ON KNEES

- Carefully move into a kneeling position, with shoulders, hips, and thighs all in line with each other and your hands hanging relaxed at your sides.
- Inhale fully as you sweep your straight arms up at the sides to reach for the ceiling above your head. Keep your back and neck in one lengthening line, so that your gaze is straight in front of you, as if you are looking toward a distant horizon.
- Sweep your straight arms down in front of you to your sides, exhaling slowly as you do so.

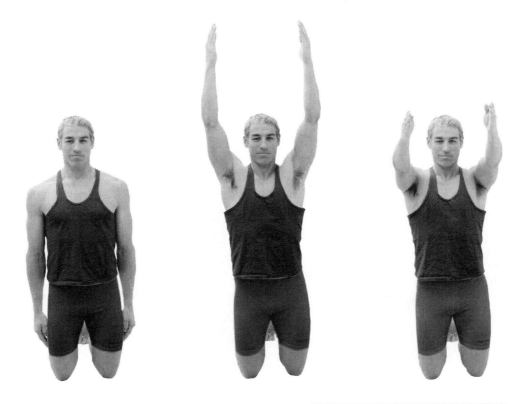

INTERMEDIATE LOCUST POSTURE

- Carefully move into a prone position, lying flat on the floor on your stomach with your legs straight and arms fully extended.

- Keeping your knees straight, raise one leg and the opposite arm off the floor as you inhale fully. It does not matter how high you raise the leg and opposite arm, as long as you keep them straight and both the knee and elbow are off the floor. Raising the opposite arm and leg together stretches the abdominal wall more fully than the Series A posture. It also engages the whole back, rather than focusing solely on the lower back.

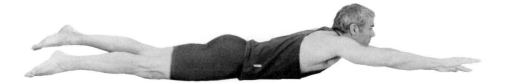

- Exhale slowly, and hold the position for six more full breaths in and out.

- Relax back to the starting position as you take an eighth breath.

- Repeat the exercise with the other leg, then do a Sun Salutation on Knees.

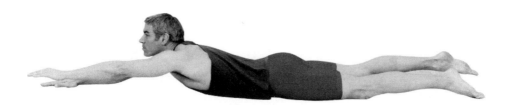

INTERMEDIATE BACK EXTENSION

- Take a position on all fours, with your weight distributed evenly on your hands and knees.
- Keep your neck and back in line with each other. Inhale fully as you lift one leg and extend it backward, and raise the opposite arm and reach forward. Try to feel your neck and back lengthening into one continuous line with the extended leg. Don't cant or tip the hip of the extended leg out of parallel with the other hip, as that will put excessive strain on the canted side.

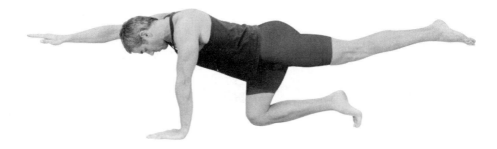

- Exhale slowly, then hold the position for six more breaths in and out.
- Relax back to the starting position on hands and knees as you take an eighth breath.
- Check to make sure your weight is once again distributed evenly on all fours, then repeat the posture by extending the other leg and arm.
- Perform a Sun Salutation on Knees.

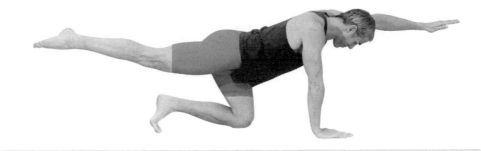

STANDING CAT STRETCH

- The Standing Cat Stretch gives you a more extended spinal stretch than the Series A Cat Stretch by working the thoracic and cervical areas of the back as well as the lumbar region. It also allows for deeper breathing that helps increase your lung capacity.

- Stand up straight with your feet about the same width apart as your shoulder blades. Keeping your back and neck as straight as possible, carefully bend forward and rest your hands on your knees.

- Curve your back into a C-shape and take seven full breaths in and out.

- Then reach for the floor in front of your feet with your belly button, and take seven more deep breaths in and out.

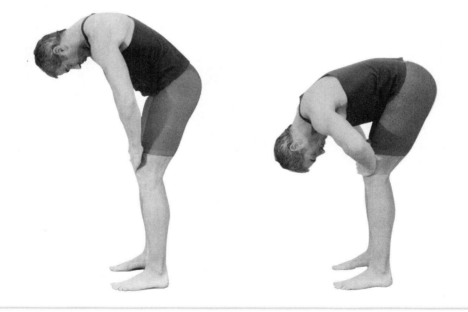

SUN SALUTATION STANDING

- Stand straight and tall with your feet together or about the same width apart as your shoulder blades, whichever is more comfortable.
- Sweep your arms up to the sides and above your head as you inhale fully.
- Sweep your straight arms down in front of you to return to rest at your sides as you exhale slowly.

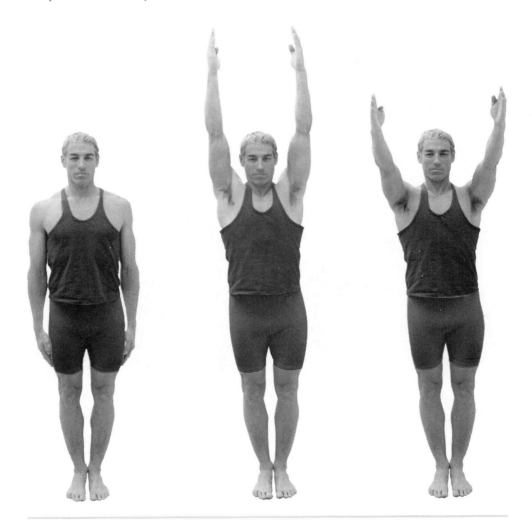

STANDING TWIST

- Stand straight and tall with your feet about the same width apart as your shoulder blades, and rest your hands on your hips. Compared to the Flexibility Prayer in Series A, this limits your shoulder turn and increases your spinal twist.
- Rotate as far as possible to one side as you inhale fully.
- Exhale slowly, then hold the position for six more deep breaths in and out.
- Relax back to the starting position as you take an eighth breath.
- Rotate to the other side, holding the position for seven full breaths in and out. Then perform a Sun Salutation Standing.

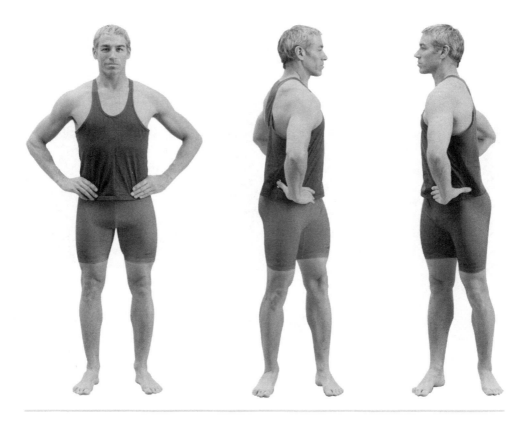

STANDING TREE POSE

- Stand straight and tall with your feet about the same width apart as your shoulder blades. Keep your neck straight so that you are looking directly in front of you, as if at a distant horizon.
- Bring the sole of one foot up to rest against the knee of the other leg.
- Inhale slowly as you raise your arms to reach for the sky.

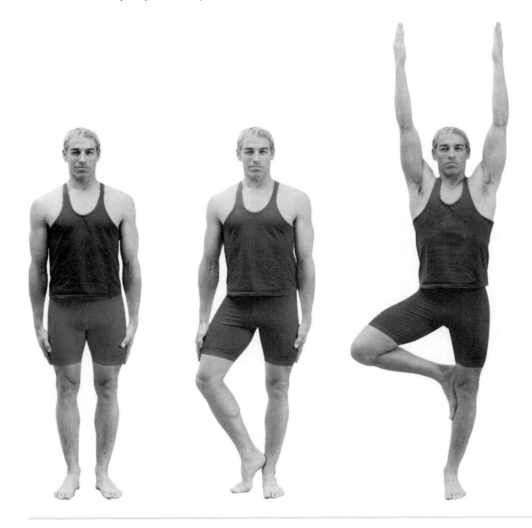

- Exhale slowly, and take six more deep breaths in and out. To maximize your proprioception, try to do this with your eyes closed.
- Relax to the starting position as you take an eighth full breath.
- Repeat on the other leg.
- Perform a Sun Salutation Standing.

You've now completed Back Rx Series B. Doing this workout consistently every day, assuming you can first do Series A totally pain-free, should bring you back to full freedom of movement and enable you to resume all your normal activities, including recreational sports, usually in about two to four weeks.

CHAPTER TEN

INTO THE FAST LANE: BACK Rx SERIES C

This demanding routine should only be started if you can do Back Rx Series B totally pain-free. It is done without Sun Salutations to set and reset a good breathing tempo, so it really works your proprioception and mind-body focus as well as your flexibility, strength, and endurance. If you're ready, it's an enormously rewarding challenge.

Series C requires you to hold each position, or to continue each movement (the greater Pilates component in Series C means much more dynamic muscle work than in Series A or B) for ten deep, full breaths in and out. This is a goal to work toward, not something you have to achieve on the first try. More difficult than holding each position or continuing each movement for ten full breaths is keeping a steady breathing flow throughout the whole routine. As you get comfortable with the routine, strive to move more and more smoothly and continuously from one exercise to another, without having to pause to catch, or reset, your breath. Series C will really build your lung capacity, which is highly important to overall health.

The whole routine should take about fifteen or twenty minutes. Once again, however, while you're doing the exercises, watch your breathing, not the clock.

THE HUNDRED

- Lie flat on your back with your knees bent, feet flat on the floor.
- Reach your hands toward your knees. The reach is from the shoulder, and your shoulders should come off the floor before your head does.
- Maintaining that extended reach from the shoulder, beat both arms down and up in parallel, keeping a strong, steady rhythm for ten full breaths in and out.
- Relax flat on your back as you take an eleventh breath.

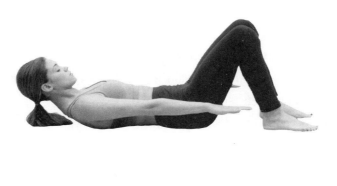

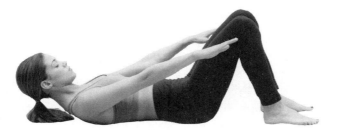

ADVANCED CRUNCH

- Lie flat on your back with your knees bent and your arms crossed over your chest.
- Bring your shoulders off the floor and gently twist one shoulder toward the opposite knee. Hold the twist for ten full breaths. This really works the internal and external obliques.
- Relax back to the starting position as you take an eleventh breath. Then bring your shoulders off the floor again and repeat the twist on the other side. Hold this counter-twist for ten full breaths (if you cannot hold the position for a full ten breaths at first, make sure to keep the number of breaths on each side consistent with the other).
- Relax back to the starting position as you take an eleventh breath.

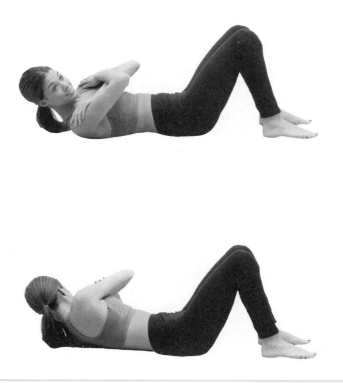

CRISS-CROSS

- Lie flat on your back with your knees bent and your hands clasped under your head. The center of your low back should remain flat on the floor for the entire exercise, as if it were glued to the floor.
- Straighten one leg, and point your toes to two o'clock, keeping your thighs parallel with each other. Pointing the toes throughout the exercise will develop a greater range of motion in the hip.
- Now get a bicycling motion going with your legs. Straighten each leg in turn as if you were trying to touch the two o'clock position with the tips of your toes. At the furthest stretch you want to have a straight line from the top of your big toe

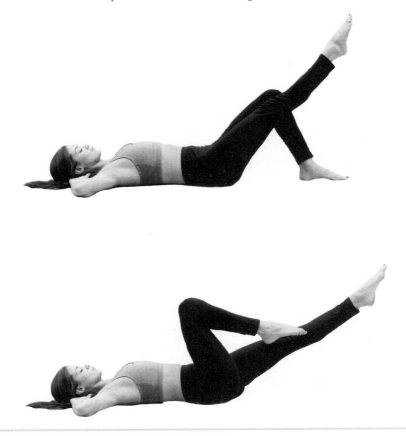

to the top of the thigh. Imagine beads of water dropping on your toe and running smoothly down that line in single file, without a single bump to interrupt or divert them.

- Keeping your shoulders straight, bring your upper body into play by alternately twisting up on each side and reaching your elbow toward your opposite knee. You should eventually be able to touch your knee with the tip of your elbow. Don't let your elbows fold in toward each other as you do this exercise; it's important to keep them fanned out as much as possible. Your elbows should stay even with your ears, so that your upper arms form a single straight line with your shoulders.

- Continue the alternating movement for ten deep, rhythmic breaths in and out.

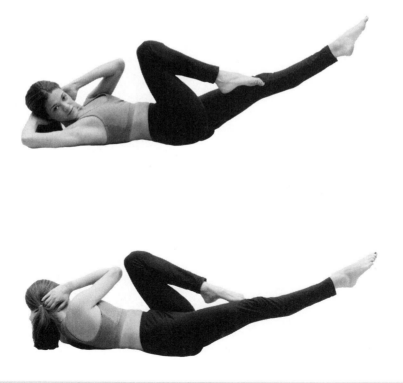

REVERSE CRUNCH

- Lie flat on your back with your arms straight and long at your sides, palms flat on the floor.
- Curl your knees up toward your chest as if you were going to roll into a reverse somersault. As your knees roll up over your chest, straighten your legs and try to touch the ceiling with the balls of your feet.

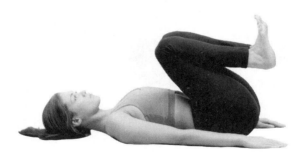

- Take ten full breaths in and out, and keep reaching for the ceiling with the balls of your feet. Your knees should remain in line with your chest.
- Relax back into a bent-knee position with your feet flat on the floor as you take an eleventh breath.

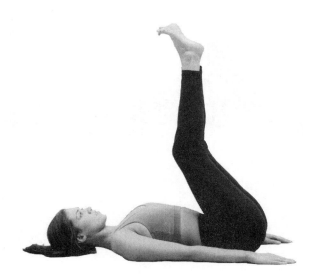

CIRCLES

- Lie flat on your back with your arms straight and long at your sides, palms flat on the floor. Stretch your legs out as long as possible, flex your feet forward, and point your toes straight ahead. Then raise one leg into a bent-knee position with your foot flat on the floor.

- Swing the bent leg up into the air and take it through as wide a circular arc as you can. Flex the foot and point your toes. This stretches the hip flexors to their maximum, developing an increased range of motion in the hip. The movement also gives a good workout to your lower abdominals and obliques.

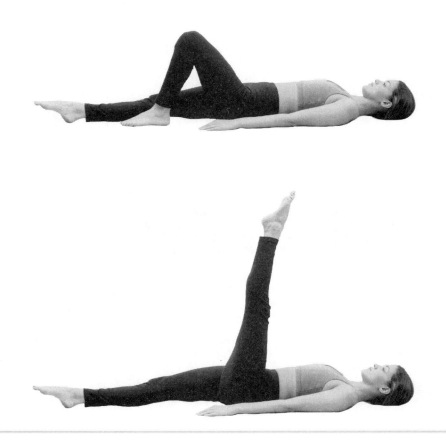

- Continue circling the leg around for ten full breaths in and out.
- Relax back to the starting position.
- Repeat the exercise with the other leg for ten full breaths in and out.

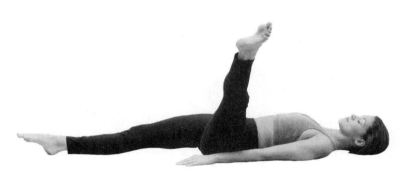

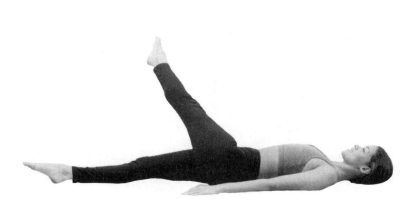

HAMSTRING STRETCH LYING DOWN

- Lie flat on your back with your arms straight and long at your sides, palms flat on the floor. Raise your knees into a bent position with your feet flat on the floor.
- Lift one leg, clasp your hands behind your knee, and pull gently.
- In this exercise, don't point your toes to the ceiling. Instead, keep the sole of your foot parallel to the floor, as if you were trying to balance a teacup on the bottom of the heel. Your shoulders should stay flat to the floor, as if they were

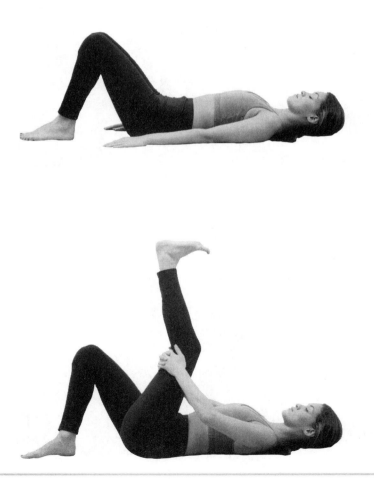

glued there, and the opposite foot should also be grounded firmly but gently, sole flat on the floor.

- Hold the stretch for ten deep breaths in and out.
- Repeat with the other leg for ten deep breaths in and out.

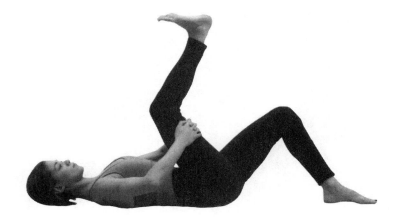

ADVANCED BRIDGING

- Lie flat on your back with your arms straight and long at your sides, palms flat on the floor, and raise your knees into a bent position.
- Straighten one leg and point your toes, keeping your thighs parallel to each other.

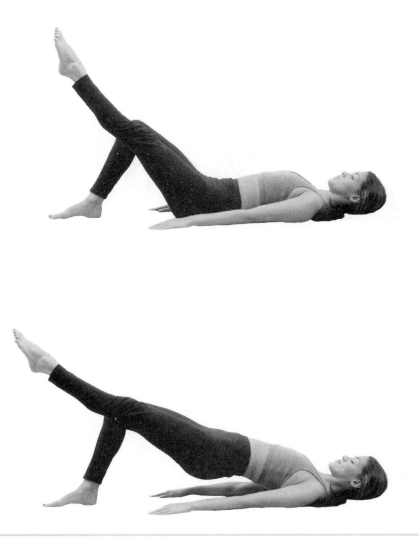

- Tighten your buttocks, pull in your abdominal muscles, and roll your hips upward until your pelvis forms a straight line with your thighs.
- Repeat with the other leg straight.

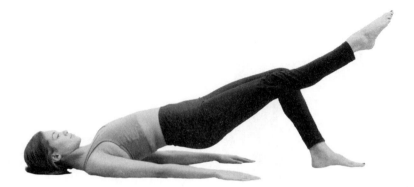

HAMSTRING STRETCH SEATED

- Sit down on the floor with your legs extended straight in front of you, toes pointed to the ceiling. Rest your palms flat on the floor beside your knees.
- Bend one leg and place the sole of that foot against the inside of your other knee. The side of the bent knee should touch the floor if possible.
- Keeping your back straight, lean forward as far as possible from the waist. As you lean forward, your chest and abdominals should lead the way, and your head,

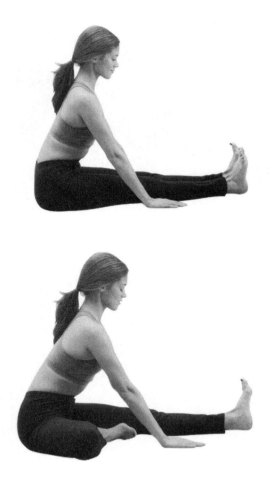

neck, and shoulders should follow. Try to keep your arms straight, too, sliding your palms forward a little as you lean into the stretch.

- Hold the stretch for ten full breaths in and out.

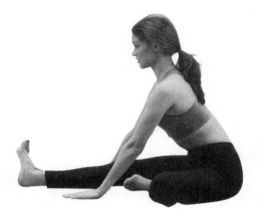

UPWARD-FACING DOG

- Lie flat on your stomach with your toes pointed straight back and your hands tucked under your shoulders.
- Feel your back and your neck forming one long line, and raise your upper body in one unit from the waist.
- Don't push up with your arms. But let them straighten and support you gently as you feel the stretch in the small of your back and your hips. Your neck should form a single line with your back, and your gaze should be straight ahead, as if

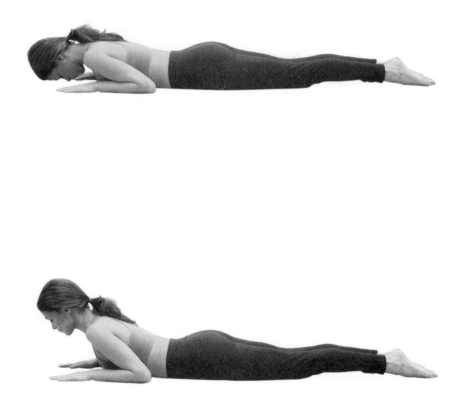

looking at a distant horizon. This keeps your neck relaxed and open to facilitate good breathing.

* Hold the position at the limit of your stretch for ten full breaths in and out.

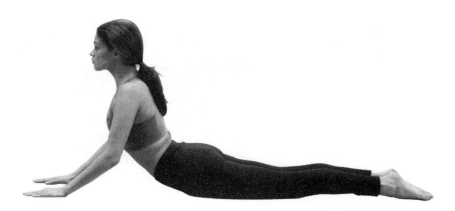

PRONE LEG BEATS

- Lie flat on your stomach with your toes pointing straight back and your hands folded underneath your chin. Your heels should be touching.
- Raise your straight knees and legs off the ground in one piece.
- As you take ten full breaths in and out, tap your heels together.

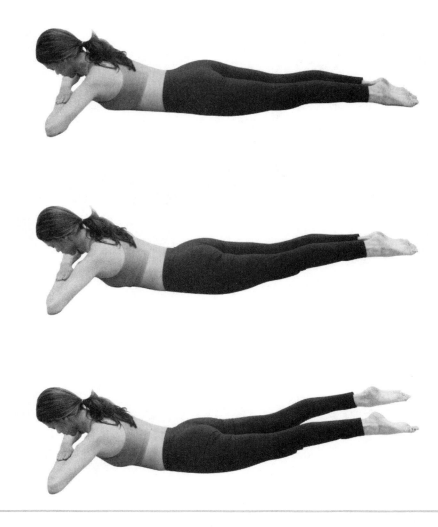

ALTERNATING SUPERMAN

- Lie on your stomach straight and long, with your toes pointed behind you and your arms extended in front of you, palms flat on the floor.
- Scissor your arms and legs at a steady, rhythmic beat for ten full breaths in and out.
- You shouldn't feel any strain in your neck. Try to keep your neck open and relaxed, so that it seems to form a continuous line with your spine.

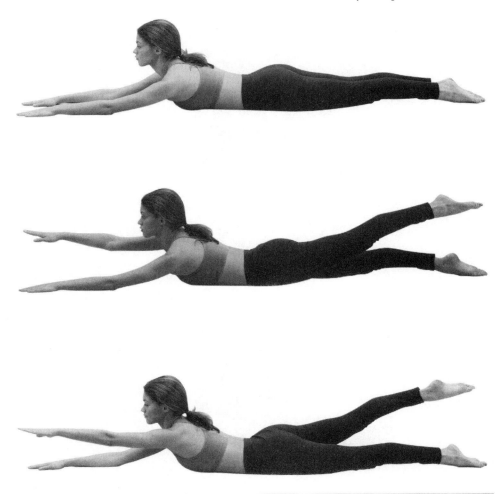

KNEE TO CHEST ON ALL FOURS

- Take a position on all fours, with your weight evenly distributed on your hands and knees.
- Arch your back into a gentle C-shape, and pull one knee toward your chest.
- Hold the knee as close to your chest as possible for ten full breaths in and out.
- Repeat with the other leg for ten full breaths in and out.

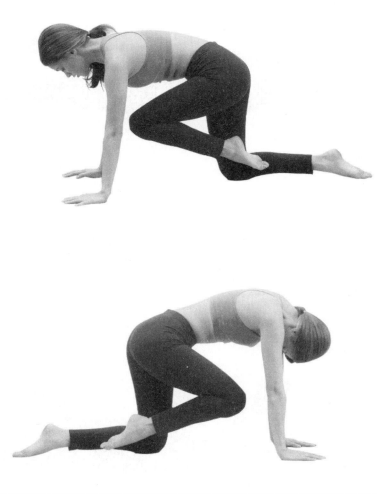

FIERCE (UNEVEN) POSTURE

- Stand up straight and tall, with your feet about the same width apart as your shoulder blades, and reach up as if you were trying to touch the ceiling with the tips of your fingers. Pigeon-toe your feet slightly, or point them straight ahead.
- Keeping your back and neck as straight as possible, sit down as if there were a chair right under you. Pretend that the seat of the chair is dropping ever so slowly to the floor, and try to catch up with it so that it can support your weight.
- This is a very simple looking posture. But the fitter you are, the more you can get out of it.

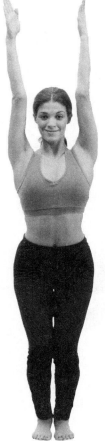

ADVANCED STANDING TREE POSE

- Stand straight and tall with your feet about the same width apart as your shoulder blades. Keep your neck straight, as if you were gazing at a distant horizon.
- Bring the sole of one foot up to rest against the knee of the other leg.
- Inhale slowly as you raise your arms to reach for the sky.
- Exhale slowly, and take nine more deep breaths in and out. To maximize your proprioception, try to do this with your eyes closed.
- Relax to the starting position as you take an eleventh full breath.
- Repeat on the other leg.

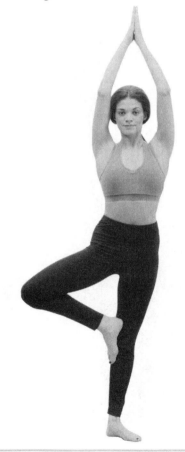

PART THREE

CHAPTER ELEVEN

OTHER CAREGIVERS

In Chapter 3 we briefly considered the other caregivers, besides general practice and specialist M.D.s, who regularly treat low back pain, including physical therapists, osteopaths, massage therapists, chiropractors, and acupunturists. Here is more information on these caregivers and their treatments to help you decide which ones may be appropriate for you in tandem with the Back Rx program.

PHYSICAL THERAPY

When physiatrists and other M.D.s write prescriptions for low back problems, physical therapy is very often the medication of choice. Because of their rigorous training in conventional medicine and the musculoskeletal system, physical therapists have a lot to offer at every stage of low back pain care. Physical therapists can diagnose and calibrate muscle imbalances, administer physical therapy, and prescribe appropriate programs of rehabilitative exercise. A physical therapist with an orthopedic specialty certificate (O.C.S.) or a doctorate in physical therapy is likely to be especially well trained to diagnose and treat low back pain.

Physical therapy is hands-on therapy, and the therapist must be someone you trust and feel comfortable with. If you find yourself ill at ease with a physical therapist, or any other medical professional for that matter, it indicates that healing will be hard to come by in that person's care. Beyond that, it's important to know that physical therapists are licensed differently in different states. Good therapists will be happy to tell you about the requirements in your state and to show you their degrees, licenses, and other certificates of training.

On your first visit to a physical therapist, you should expect the therapist to take a thorough medical history and do a careful assessment of your muscle strength and range of motion, especially in the hips. As the therapist examines and treats you, he or she should explain each procedure and the sensations you will likely feel. With a capable therapist you should very rarely be surprised by sharp pain and never experience repeated sharp pain.

Many techniques of physical therapy have something in common with those of medical massage, osteopathy, and chiropractic. But because each form of therapy practices from a different perspective and knowledge base, the effect and the experience of each can be vastly different. There can also be great differences among different therapists' versions of the same treatment. When you are looking for a caregiver, word-of-mouth recommendations from people you trust can give you a sense of the subjective differences between one treatment, or one practitioner, and another.

OSTEOPATHY

Osteopathic medical school provides rigorous, high-level education and training in all aspects of human health. In 1999 the *New England Journal of Medicine* reported that osteopathy has been proven effective for low back pain in controlled clinical trials.

From a theoretical point of view, osteopathy sees the body as a self-healing mechanism and accordingly puts great emphasis on proper patient exercise, rest, and nutrition. Brian Waldron, D.O. (Doctor of Osteopathy), a leading osteopathic physician and professor of osteopathic medicine at the New York College of Osteopathy, says that when it comes to low back pain in particular, "The rehab work a patient does is really the glue that holds the healing together."

To facilitate rehabilitation and unblock the body's self-recuperative powers, osteopathy offers low back sufferers a set of gentle, unhurried, hands-on techniques, including medical massage and physical therapy-like manipulations. In treating disc-related low back pain, osteopathic physicians look for structural asymmetries and points of counterstrain, like a pelvic twist that leads to misalignment of the spinal facet joints. They then try to correct the asymmetries and relieve the counterstrain with direct, but usually very subtle and gentle manipulations such as a High Velocity/Low Amplitude Thrust. The procedure sounds scary, but really isn't. The technique is High Velocity because it is quick, like the blink of an eye. But the force behind the thrust is very gentle, and thus Low Amplitude.

Like a physical therapist, an osteopathic physician should explain procedures along the way and prepare you for the sensations that the treatment is likely to evoke.

MASSAGE THERAPY

Medical massage, which I discussed at length in Chapter 3, is the only other alternative, or integrated, therapy besides osteopathy to be proven effective for low back pain in controlled clinical trials. In 2001, the *Annals of Internal Medicine* reported that massage therapy had passed this stringent test.

I have seen many patients derive great benefit from massage therapy, especially in tandem with Back Rx and similar rehabilitative exercises. It can often quickly short-circuit a low back pain cycle and provide the respite your body needs to begin healing properly.

CHIROPRACTIC

Chiropractic is another form of treatment that can be beneficial for low back pain. Chiropractors have long had a "snap, crackle, and pop" reputation for dramatic, and perhaps excessively forceful, spinal and cervical manipulations. This criticism has probably never been fair to the vast majority of chiropractors. And it has lost much of its accuracy over the last twenty years, according to my colleague Carol Goldstein, D.C. (Doctor of Chiropractic), as a generational shift in chiropractic education, training, and practice has taken place.

Chiropractic aims to diagnose and treat low back pain by identifying and correcting soft tissue irregularities, neuromuscular imbalances, and skeletal misalignments. Although these treatment practices use many similar techniques, it is fair to say that chiropractic manipulations still tend to be more forceful, on average, than those of osteopathy, physical therapy, or massage therapy. In this regard, much depends on the individual chiropractor.

"The more refined your technique, the less force you need to use," Dr. Goldstein points out. She has helped many of my patients with her skill in gentle manipulations combined with the healing touch. Chiropractors should always explain the treatment they are giving, and prepare you for the physical sensations you will experience while receiving it. I would only repeat my caution from Chapter 3, that you not undergo any high-velocity manipulations of the head and neck, because in rare cases they can trigger strokes. The risk may be slight, but I don't think it's worth taking.

The experiences of many patients testify to chiropractic's potential to aid healing in significant ways. I don't hesitate to recommend chiropractic care under reputable chiropractors for those patients who seem well suited to it.

ACUPUNCTURE

Acupuncture is the ancient practice of stimulating specific points—called "acu-points"—a few centimeters beneath the surface of the skin with fine, solid metal needles that are considerably smaller than the hypodermic needles used for injections. An acupuncturist may stimulate the acupoints by manipulating the needles gently, heating them with burning herbs (known as moxibustion), or running a mild electric current through them. Traditional Chinese medicine locates acupoints along meridians, which are pathways for the flow of vital energy, or qi (pronounced "chee"), within the body. The meridians connect the nervous system with other parts of the body.

Acupuncture for treating back pain may be 5,000 years old. The "Tyrolean ice man" discovered in a glacier in the Alps in 1991 dates to that period, and the scientists who examined his body found both that he had significant back arthritis and that he had tattoos on the inside of the heel and along the Achilles tendon exactly where traditional Chinese medicine locates acupoints for the back.

In modern China, acupuncture continues to be used frequently as an anesthetic in all sorts of operations. The pain blocking mechanism of acupuncture is not yet fully understood, but its effects have been demonstrated in many studies. As yet there has been no controlled clinical trial of acupuncture in low back pain, but in 1997 the National Institutes of Health termed acupuncture a safe, viable treatment for low back pain, osteoarthritis, tennis elbow, carpal tunnel syndrome, fibromyalgia, nausea from chemotherapy, post-operative pain, nausea during pregnancy, and menstrual cramps.

Some people very much enjoy receiving acupuncture and say that it promotes relaxation and a feeling of well-being. Other people have an aversion to needles. But you can be confident that acupuncture is safe when performed by a skilled acupuncturist, who may be a practitioner of traditional Chinese medicine or an

M.D. who has also been trained and licensed in acupuncture. In either case, the person performing acupuncture should use only disposable needles. As with other caregivers, the best way to find a good acupuncturist is through trusted word-of-mouth recommendations.

Both acute and chronic low back pain cases may respond well to acupuncture. According to my colleague Robert Schulman, M.D., L. Ac. (Licensed Acupuncturist), acute cases of low back pain can usually be resolved with two to three sessions of acupuncture. Chronic cases may require a short or long course of treatment to end the pain, with most patients finding six-plus sessions over the span of a few weeks effective.

All the treatments and therapies discussed in this chapter are appropriate for Stage I care (see Chapter 3). When used along with Back Rx or a similar program of rehabilitative exercise, they can help the vast majority of low back pain sufferers to achieve a full and lasting recovery. For the minority of patients who need more help to heal, conventional medicine now offers a number of innovative, non-invasive, nonsurgical treatments, as well as ways to minimize the trauma of surgery. Chapter 3 gives an overview of these state-of-the-art procedures; to close the book, I'd like to tell you about the differences I've seen them make in patients' lives.

CHAPTER TWELVE

STATE-OF-THE-ART TREATMENTS AND THE FUTURE OF LOW BACK CARE

As discussed in Chapter 3, most low back pain sufferers can achieve a full recovery with Stage I care, but a minority of low back pain patients, perhaps 20% or fewer, require treatments from Stage II, III, or IV care. These treatments are the fruit of ongoing research and clinical innovation in conventional medicine, which has made it possible to localize pain sources far more precisely than ever before and deliver medicine to those exact areas.

From midlife on, low back pain treatment is increasingly complicated by the fact that there may be multiple generators of pain in a herniated disc itself, the spinal vertebrae, and the facet and sacroiliac (SI) joints (see Chapter 1, Figures 1 and 2). Using fluoroscopy (X-ray guidance), physicians can now sort out which of these areas is the primary source of the pain. As a rule of thumb, these procedures generally show that increased back and leg pain from sitting can be traced to the discs, whereas increased pain from standing and walking tends to center on the facet and SI joints and to age-related narrowing of the spinal column known as spinal stenosis.

Except where noted below, Stage II and later treatments should be combined with Back Rx or a similar exercise program.

STAGE II TREATMENTS:
TRIGGER POINT AND GUIDED EPIDURAL AND FACET INJECTIONS

If you have severe ongoing back pain but no leg symptoms from a herniated disc that fails to respond to Stage I care, you are a candidate for paravertebral, or trigger point, injections of a saline solution. The trigger points are those areas where you feel the most discomfort. These injections can be very effective at controlling low back pain if two or three of them are done a couple of weeks apart. Each procedure takes about five minutes in the doctor's office.

If you have leg symptoms as well as persistent, severe back pain from a herniated disc, you are a candidate for a selective nerve-root epidural under fluoroscopy, also known as a guided epidural. This fifteen- to twenty-minute procedure delivers a precisely measured dose of lidocaine and corticosteroid directly to the inflamed nerve that is the source of the pain, as determined with the aid of fluoroscopy. The nerve may be inflamed because a disc protrusion is impinging on it. Or it may be inflamed by leaking disc fluid, which is toxic to the surrounding tissues, a condition known as chemical radiculitis.

I have had an opportunity to help innovate this procedure, and in an article in the January 2002 issue of the journal *Spine*, my colleagues and I report an 84% success rate when combined with rehabilitative exercise. That is, 84% of those who received the injections in our study and who then completed Back Rx were pain-free a year later. And there were no complications as a result of the injections.

Just one of these injections can bring about a dramatic change in healing, as I saw with a patient one Friday. A corporate road warrior and working mother in her mid-thirties, in good overall health and not overweight, Mary G. had just crawled in from JFK Airport and a nonstop flight from Tokyo, which she had only survived thanks to the fortifying effects of a bottle of Burgundy. Forty-eight hours before, she had landed at Narita Airport outside Tokyo on a business trip. Reaching down to pull her checked bag off the carousel, Mary felt something pop in her back and dropped to the floor in pain. She was taken to a local hospital, where she was advised that surgery was necessary to remove a herniated disc protrusion.

Imagine being on your own in a foreign country where you don't speak the language and having to make that kind of decision about your health. Mary called a friend in New York who happened to be one of my patients, and the upshot of that was her arrival at the Hospital for Special Surgery, where the nurses kindly kept the treatment room open late for her.

When Mary finally reached the hospital a little after 5:00 PM, I wondered if she had flown all that way in agony for nothing. She was completely hunched over in pain and could barely stumble a few steps at a time with assistance. Twenty minutes later, however, after receiving a single guided epidural injection under local anesthesia, she got up off the treatment table pain-free and was able to go home and give her child a hug without any stress or strain. With the pain cycle broken, she was also able to begin Back Rx and heal without surgery.

Similar injections can be done of the facet and SI joints, if X rays show that they are the source of the pain. But injection of the facet and SI joints tends to be much less successful, providing long-term relief to only about 50% of the patients who receive them.

STAGE III TREATMENTS:
RADIO FREQUENCY DENERVATION, MICRO-DISCECTOMY, LAMINECTOMY, IDET, AND NUCLEOPLASTY

If you have pain in the facet and SI joints that does not respond to Stage II treatment, a procedure called Radio Frequency Denervation has been shown to be very effective. A 2001 study in *Spine* reported that 80% of patients remained pain-free a year after undergoing this fluoroscopically guided procedure, in which a tiny probe is used to heat the small nerves that innervate the facet or SI joints. This halts the pain by making the nerves inactive for a couple of years, after which time the procedure can be done again.

My colleagues at the Hospital for Special Surgery and I studied the effectiveness of Radio Frequency Denervation in twelve baseball pitchers with inflamed facet joints. Nine of the twelve were professional baseball players, and the other three were collegiate players. After the procedure, eleven of the twelve were able to resume pitching competitively.

My patient Jesse G. also benefited greatly from Radio Frequency Denervation. An eighty-year-old business executive, Jesse was hunched forward in a wheelchair when he came to see me. He had severe right-sided low back and buttock pain, and he could barely walk half a block without assistance. He had a history of laminectomies (see below) going back about twenty years, and pronounced spinal stenosis and arthritis. Through X rays and physical examination we determined that the majority of his pain was coming from the right-sided facet joints. We did Radio Frequency Denervation on those joints, with the result that Jesse's pain decreased 60–70%, his posture improved, and he was able to walk five to seven blocks at a time. He still wasn't pain-free by any means, but his quality of life improved tremendously. Although Jesse was too debilitated for Back Rx, wearing a cryobrace (a back brace that holds an ice pack) twice a day and aquatherapy enabled him to maintain the gains from the radio frequency heating of his facet joints.

If you have a large herniated disc with back and leg pain, and Stage II care fails to stop the pain, you are a candidate for a micro-discectomy or a laminectomy. Patients with both back and leg pain experience an 85% cure rate with these procedures. Patients with back pain alone have much lower success rates.

People who form scar tissue easily should let their doctors know about this before having a micro-discectomy or laminectomy. If you find that even small cuts tend to heal slowly and wind up covered with smooth, shiny, slightly pink patches of skin, you may be in this group. These patches of shiny skin are fibrous tissues called keloids ("key-loids"), which can seriously complicate the healing of surgical wounds.

If you have back pain alone that *increases* with sitting and your MRI shows disc pathology, a discogram can help determine the source of the pain. In a discogram, dye is injected at different disc levels so that it becomes possible to tell precisely which levels are causing pain. After the discogram, a CT or CAT (Computed Tomography or Computer Aided Tomography) scan is also done to provide a look at the structure of the discs. If the discogram and the CAT scan both point to the same disc levels, the discogram is said to be positive. If these tests also localize the problem down to only one or two disc levels, you become a candidate for disc heating. The procedure is not appropriate when more disc levels are involved. It is also inappropriate if the discogram is negative.

There are two forms of disc heating. If a patient has a positive discogram with a tear in the annulus, the hard outer portion of the disc, a disc heating procedure called Intradiscal Electrothermal Therapy (IDET) can be performed. In this procedure an electrode is wrapped around the annulus to heat it. The heat stiffens the disc, seals cracks, and desensitizes nerve endings. The procedure takes about an hour under fluoroscopy and studies have shown that it provides the majority of patients who have it with good or excellent pain relief.

If the discogram is positive and there is a contained disc protrusion without an annular tear, a nucleoplasty can be done. A nucleoplasty heats the inner portion of the disc, the nucleus pulposus, rather than the annulus, and has a similarly good success rate. The procedure takes about half an hour to perform.

Disc heating has made the difference in many of my patients' recoveries from low back pain. One of those it has helped is Rick G., a special ed teacher. Rick was twenty-seven when I first examined him, a fit, healthy young man who worked out regularly. One day at school an agitated child yanked on his arm. Rick heard a pop in his back, he collapsed in pain, and he was bedridden for a week. Chiropractic therapy, acupuncture, oral medications, and epidural injections all failed to help him. His doctors told him there was nothing left to try but a fusion. Then he came to see me.

Rick had severe localized low back pain, but no leg symptoms. His MRI showed a contained central disc protrusion at L4–L5. I told him about nucleoplasty, including the drawback it shares with IDET, namely that it may slightly increase the degeneration of a disc, and Rick decided to give it a try.

Most people will not experience pain relief from a nucleoplasty until six to eight weeks after the procedure. But some patients receive immediate relief. Rick was one of them. He got up off the treatment table after the thirty-minute procedure and said, "What happened? My pain is gone." He was then able to return to work, and eventually to begin Back Rx in order to strengthen his back and prevent recurrences.

After an IDET or nucleoplasty, the heated disc is temporarily susceptible to micro-instability. To protect the disc it is necessary to wear a back brace for eight weeks, and to receive physical therapy and aquatherapy, before going on to something like Back Rx.

STAGE IV TREATMENTS:
DISC REPLACEMENT AND SPINAL FUSION

If you have severe disc degeneration at one or two levels, but not more, you will, in the near future, be a candidate for artificial disc replacement. Replacement discs are now being studied in FDA trials, and they should be approved for wide use in two or three years.

If disc degeneration is more widespread, a CT myelogram (a scan with dye) can provide a detailed road map of the anatomy to help determine whether or not to perform a spinal fusion, either endoscopic or open. In an open fusion surgeons make a long incision in the back and then peel back layers of muscle to expose the spine, remove the herniated or degenerated disc or disc portion, and lock the vertebrae on either side together with a small metal pin or bracket. In an endoscopic fusion, surgeons use a fiber-optic viewing tube (the endoscope) and other instruments to operate through one or two small holes in the back. Although it is much less traumatic than an open fusion, an endoscopic fusion still requires a fairly lengthy recovery period.

As with a micro-discectomy or laminectomy, people who form scar tissue easily should alert their doctors before a fusion is performed. Post-surgical scars can scuttle any good the fusion achieves.

Back fusions, whether open or endoscopic, have a less than 50% success rate for people with severe back pain but no leg pain. But there is a more than 90% success rate for fusions in people who have back and leg pain with severe stenosis (narrowing of the spinal column) and spondylolisthesis, in which the bones of the spine slip on top of each other.

THE FUTURE OF LOW BACK CARE

Current medical research promises potential low back care breakthroughs on two fronts. First, because chemical radiculitis (inflammation from leaking disc fluid), rather than actual impingement of a disc fragment on a nerve, is often the chief source of pain in disc herniations and tears, researchers are investigating whether injecting growth factors and anti-inflammatories directly into the disc can neutralize the inflammatory chemicals it contains and thus halt the disc's pain and degeneration. Second, gene therapy techniques are being used to try to turn on cells that can reproduce an injured nucleus pulposus in pristine shape.

It's too soon to tell for sure, but my hunch is that the research in these areas is far enough along to make one or both of these therapies available in the relatively near future, perhaps within the next decade. Whatever the future brings, however, Back Rx or a similar program will remain the front line of treatment for low back problems. Nothing else is so time- and cost-effective at restoring and sustaining back health. Because of its unsurpassed ability to speed the healing of low back problems and minimize and prevent recurrences, Back Rx will always be one of the very best things you can do for your back.

APPENDIX:
RESOURCES ON THE WEB

- Medline Plus Health Information, a service of the U.S. National Library of Medicine (NLM) and the National Institutes of Health (NIH), has state-of-the-art information on all medical matters, including low back pain: *www.nlm.nih.gov/medlineplus/* or *www.nlm.nih.gov*
- American Association of Neurological Surgeons: *www.aans.org*
- American Academy of Orthopaedic Surgeons: *www.aaos.org*
- International Spinal Injection Society fosters techniques for precision diagnosis of spinal pain: *www.spinalinjection.com*
- North American Spine Society: *www.spine.org*
- American Academy of Physical Medicine and Rehabilitation: *www.aapmr.org*

INTEGRATED CARE

- National Center for Complementary and Alternative Medicine, part of the NIH, offers information on acupuncture and other forms of integrated care: *www.nccam.nih.gov*